Handbook of Pharmacovigilance

Principles, Practice and Global Drug Safety

A JULLIYAN DILLEBAN

NOTION PRESS

Dedicated to

Almighty

&

My Respected Parents

Foreword

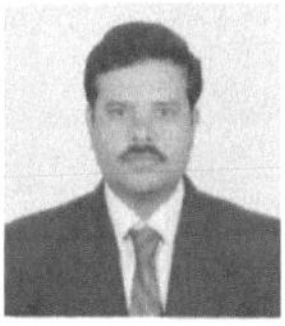

Drug safety is a major concern in healthcare. Every day, millions of people worldwide take medications to treat illnesses and improve their health. However, not all medicines are risk-free. Pharmacovigilance, the practice of monitoring and evaluating the safety of drugs, plays a vital role in protecting patients and ensuring that medications are safe and effective.

In this context, Dr. Julliyan Dilleban's handbook on pharmacovigilance is a timely and invaluable contribution. The author combines academic precision with practical clarity, bridging the gap between theory and real-world applications. This comprehensive guide offers essential knowledge on identifying and reporting adverse drug reactions, understanding international drug safety frameworks.

This handbook is more than a reference; it is a resource for professional growth. It encourages academicians, healthcare professionals, and students to actively participate in the global effort to promote safe medication use. I strongly believe that this work will inspire readers to uphold the highest standards of patient care and improve drug safety across healthcare systems.

Prof. Dr. N. Venkateshan, M.Pharm., Ph.D.,
Principal,
Arulmigu Kalasalingam College of Pharmacy,
Srivilliputtur, Tamil Nadu, India.

Foreword

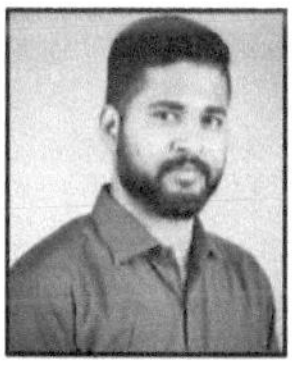

Pharmacovigilance has emerged as one of the most critical pillars of modern healthcare, ensuring that the benefits of medicines and vaccines are maximized while their risks are carefully monitored and managed. In today's era of rapid drug development, globalized clinical trials, and expanding therapeutic options, safeguarding patient safety is not merely a regulatory requirement - it is both a moral and scientific imperative.

This handbook on Pharmacovigilance has been thoughtfully compiled to serve as a comprehensive guide for students, researchers, healthcare professionals, and regulatory authorities. It provides a structured exploration of the discipline, beginning with an introduction to pharmacovigilance and adverse drug reactions (ADR), essential terminologies, drug and disease classification, and the use of drug dictionaries and coding systems. This handbook aims to empower its readers with the knowledge and tools necessary to uphold drug safety. It is not only a reference but also a call to action - a reminder that pharmacovigilance is a shared responsibility, vital to protecting lives and fostering trust in healthcare systems worldwide.

I commend the author for his dedication in creating this resource and trust that it will serve as a valuable companion for all those committed to advancing patient safety.

Dr Alan James. MBBS. MD (FM). DNB(FM).,
- **Police Surgeon & Assistant Professor,**
Department of Forensic Medicine,
Kanyakumari Government Medical College,
Asaripallam.
- **Vice Chairman,**
Sigma College of Architecture & Planning,
Moododu, Kanyakumari district.

Foreword

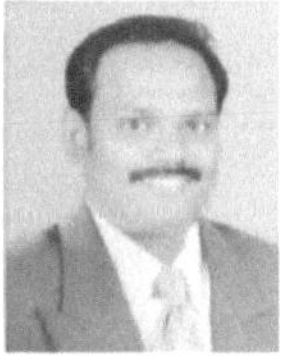

As a physiotherapist, my primary clinical focus is restoring human movement and functional independence. However, the path to physical rehabilitation is rarely isolated from medical management. The patients we treat in clinics and hospitals frequently rely on complex pharmacological support - ranging from analgesics and muscle relaxants to systemic anti-inflammatories - to tolerate therapy and heal effectively. Consequently, recognizing when a patient's sudden dizziness, profound fatigue, or unexpected muscular weakness is actually an Adverse Drug Reaction (ADR) rather than a musculoskeletal symptom is a vital clinical skill. Pharmacovigilance is not just a regulatory duty; it is a cornerstone of frontline patient care.

In the Handbook of Pharmacovigilance, Dr. A. Julliyan Dilleban has masterfully bridged the gap between complex regulatory science and practical clinical application. By meticulously detailing the fundamental concepts of drug safety - from the historical context and evolution of global monitoring practices to the intricate methodologies of causality assessment for adverse reactions - this text transforms a dense subject into highly accessible knowledge.

It is my great honor to introduce this work. I am confident that this handbook will serve as a foundational text for professionals across the healthcare spectrum, ultimately advancing our shared goal: safeguarding the health and well-being of the patients we serve.

Dr. M. Periyanayagaswamy MPT (Cardio), MIAP.,
People Forum of India, Secretary, Tamil Nadu State,
Bone and Joint Physiotherapy & Diagnostic Centre,
Neyveli, Cuddalore District, Tamil Nadu.

Preface

Pharmacovigilance has become an essential pillar of modern healthcare, ensuring that the benefits of medicines consistently outweigh their associated risks. As pharma innovation accelerates - driven by rapid drug discovery, globalized clinical trials, and expanding access to therapeutic options - the need for systematic, scientifically robust drug safety monitoring has never been more pressing. Adverse drug reactions, whether predictable or unforeseen, can only be effectively managed when healthcare systems are supported by well-designed pharmacovigilance structures and informed professionals who fully understand how these systems function.

This Handbook of Pharmacovigilance offers a concise, accessible introduction to core concepts and principles of drug safety. It covers the historical evolution of pharmacovigilance, regulatory frameworks, signal detection and risk assessment methods, and risk communication essentials. Designed to bridge technical literature and practical needs, it provides a clear pathway for learners and early-career professionals.

This handbook is primarily intended for pharmacy and healthcare students beginning their journey into pharmacovigilance. It will also prove invaluable for novice researchers and professionals working in regulatory affairs, clinical research, pharmacovigilance units, and public health organizations, as well as experienced practitioners seeking a concise refresher on key concepts. By engaging with this handbook, readers will gain a comprehensive overview of pharmacovigilance systems, the importance of adverse event reporting, the fundamentals of risk management.

I extend my sincere gratitude to Prof. Dr. N. Venkateshan, Principal of Arulmigu Kalasalingam College of Pharmacy, for his unwavering encouragement and support. Thanks to the institution for its conducive academic environment. Above all, I am profoundly thankful to my family for their enduring belief in me

Julliyan Dilleban

Glossary of Terminologies

A

Absolute risk

Probability of an event occurring in a defined population of exposed persons over a specified period, usually expressed as the number of individuals who experience the event divided by the number at risk in that group.

Adverse event (AE)

Any unfavourable and unintended sign, symptom, or disease temporally associated with the use of a medicinal product, whether or not it is considered related causally to that product.

Adverse drug reaction (ADR)

A noxious and unintended response to a medicinal product for which at least a reasonable possibility of causal relationship is suspected, including reactions arising from authorized or unauthorized use (such as off-label use, overdose, misuse, abuse, medication errors, or occupational exposure).

Allopathy

A system of medical practice that treats disease by the use of remedies (often synthetic or purified active substances) which produce effects different from, or opposing, those produced by the disease itself; in pharmacovigilance glossaries this term is used to distinguish conventional Western medicine from traditional or alternative systems.

Annual Safety Report (ASR)

A periodic report summarizing and evaluating safety information collected for an investigational or marketed product over one year, prepared to support ongoing safety oversight by sponsors and regulators (conceptually aligned with annual safety updates/DSUR for clinical trials and PSUR/PBRER for marketed products).

Archiving

The controlled retention and protection of essential pharmacovigilance and clinical trial documents for the period required by regulation or guidance so that they can be retrieved for audits, inspections, or re evaluation of safety data.

Audit

A systematic and independent examination of trialor pharmacovigilance related activities and documents to determine whether they were conducted, recorded, and reported in accordance with the protocol, standard operating procedures, Good Clinical Practice, and applicable regulatory requirements.

Attributable risk (risk difference)

The difference in the incidence (or absolute risk) of an outcome between an exposed group and a comparable unexposed (reference) group, representing the amount of risk that can be attributed to the exposure.

B

Biological products

Medicinal products whose active substances are derived from or produced by biological sources (for example, blood products, vaccines, recombinant proteins, monoclonal antibodies, or other materials of human, animal or microbiological origin).

Blinding / Masking

A procedure in which one or more parties involved in a clinical trial (such as subjects, investigators, monitors, or data analysts) are kept unaware of which treatment has been assigned, in order to reduce bias; “single blind” usually masks subjects only, and “double blind” usually masks subjects and key trial staff.

C

Causality assessment

A structured evaluation of the likelihood that a medicinal product was a contributing cause of an observed adverse event in a particular case, typically using standardized algorithms or expert judgment categories such as certain, probable, possible, unlikely, or unrelated.

Causal relationship

A judged or demonstrated cause and effect link between administration of a medicinal product and occurrence of an event, usually expressed by stating that the product is at least reasonably possibly related to the event.

Company Core Data Sheet (CCDS)

The company's reference document for a product, prepared by the marketing authorization holder, that consolidates authoritative information such as indications, dosing, pharmacology, and safety, and serves as the basis for local product information globally.

Company Core Safety Information (CCSI)

The subset of safety information in the CCDS that the marketing authorization holder designates as core safety content to be reflected in all local product information, unless modified by specific regulatory requirements.

CemFlow

A software application provided by the Uppsala Monitoring Centre to support data collection and analysis for cohort event monitoring schemes.

Challenge

(Within dechallenge–rechallenge methodology) administration of a suspect medicinal product to a patient, usually after a prior exposure, in order to observe whether an adverse event appears or recurs and thereby contribute to causality assessment.

CIOMS

The Council for International Organizations of Medical Sciences, an organization established under WHO and UNESCO that develops internationally influential guidance on ethics, pharmacovigilance, and drug development, including cumulative pharmacovigilance glossaries and working group reports.

Contract research organisation (CRO)

A person or organisation (commercial, academic, or other) contracted by a sponsor to perform one or more of the sponsor's trial related or pharmacovigilance related duties and functions.

Clinical trial

Any investigation in human subjects intended to discover or verify the clinical, pharmacological, or pharmacodynamic effects of an investigational product, identify adverse reactions, or study absorption, distribution, metabolism, and excretion, with the objective of determining its safety and/or efficacy.

Cohort event monitoring (CEM)

A prospective observational method in which a defined cohort of patients starting a specific medicine is followed systematically for a period, and all medical events are collected, in order to characterize that medicine's safety profile under real world conditions.

Compliance

The extent to which a patient's behaviour in taking medicines, following diets, or executing lifestyle changes corresponds with agreed recommendations from a healthcare provider; in trials this often refers to adherence to the dosing regimen.

Control group

The group in a clinical trial or epidemiological study that does not receive the test intervention and is used as a benchmark (for example, placebo or active comparator) against which the outcomes in the treated group are compared.

D

Data lock point (data cut off date)

The calendar date selected as the cut off for including data in a periodic safety report such as a PSUR or PBRER, often based on the product's international birth date and occurring at defined intervals (for example, every six or twelve months).

Data-mining

The use of automated statistical tools to screen large safety databases (such as VigiBase) for drug–event combinations reported more often than expected, for example with Bayesian methods like the BCPNN, to support signal detection.

Dechallenge

The withdrawal, reduction, or interruption of a suspected medicinal product to observe whether an adverse event abates or disappears, used as part of causality assessment.

Development Safety Update Report (DSUR)

A periodic safety report that provides a comprehensive, yearly assessment of the safety of an investigational drug under study in clinical trials, analogous to the PSUR/PBRER for marketed medicines.

Drug

Any substance or combination of substances presented as having properties for treating or preventing disease or that may be used or administered to diagnose, restore, correct, or modify physiological functions.

E

Effectiveness/Risk

A concept describing how well a medicine works in routine clinical practice (effectiveness) in relation to the probability and seriousness of harms it may cause (risk), forming part of overall benefit–risk evaluation.

Efficacy

The extent to which a medicinal product produces a beneficial result under ideal, controlled conditions such as randomized clinical trials.

Epidemiology

The study of the distribution and determinants of health-related states or events in specified populations, and the application of this study to control health problems.

Essential Medicines

Medicines that satisfy the priority health-care needs of the population, selected based on public-health relevance, evidence on efficacy and safety, and comparative cost-effectiveness.

EudraVigilance

The European Union system for managing and analyzing information on suspected adverse reactions to medicines authorized or being studied in the EEA, supporting electronic exchange and scientific evaluation of ICSRs.

F

Formulary

A list of medicinal products, usually with information on indications, dosage, method of administration, and restrictions, that are approved for use within a particular institution, system, or country.

G

Generic (multisource product)

A medicinal product containing the same active substance(s) as an originator (innovator) product, intended to be interchangeable with it, usually marketed after patent or exclusivity expiry and often identified by the international non-proprietary name.

H

Harm

The nature and extent of actual damage or injury that may be caused by a medicine, including physical, psychological or social impact; distinct from the probability of that damage (risk).

Herbal medicines

Medicinal products that contain, as active ingredients, herbal substances or herbal preparations derived from plants or plant parts, used for therapeutic, prophylactic or diagnostic purposes.

I

ICH

The International Council for Harmonisation of Technical Requirements for Pharmaceuticals for Human Use, a body that brings together regulatory authorities and industry to develop harmonised guidelines on drug development, safety and quality.

Information component (IC)

A Bayesian disproportionality measure used in global pharmacovigilance databases to identify drug–event combinations reported more often than expected; a positive IC value suggests higher-than-expected reporting frequency.

Incidence

The number of new cases of a disease or event occurring in a specified population during a defined period, typically expressed as a rate (e.g. cases per person-time).

Individual case safety report

A structured report that describes a suspected adverse reaction in an individual patient associated with one or more medicinal products, forming the basic unit of data in pharmacovigilance systems.

International Birth Date (IBD)

The date of first marketing authorisation for a medicinal product in any country in the world, used as the reference point for scheduling periodic safety reports.

L

Life-threatening adverse drug experience

An adverse experience which, in the view of the initial reporter, places the patient at immediate risk of death as the event occurs, not including events which might have caused death had they been more severe.

M

MedDRA

MedDRA (Medical Dictionary for Regulatory Activities) is a clinically validated, standardised international medical terminology developed by ICH and used by regulators and industry for coding, retrieval, evaluation and presentation of safety and clinical data throughout the product life cycle.

Medical error

An unintended act (either of omission or commission) or a process that does not achieve its intended outcome in the context of healthcare delivery, including prescribing, dispensing or administering medicines.

N

National Pharmacovigilance centres

Government-recognized organisations, usually within the medicines regulatory authority or designated institutions, responsible at national level for collecting, managing, analysing and communicating information on the safety of medicines.

O

Omega (Ω)

A statistical measure of disproportionality developed for detecting potential drug–drug–event interaction signals in large safety databases, comparing observed with expected reports for specific triplets.

OTC (Over the Counter) medicine

A medicinal product that can be obtained by consumers without a prescription, subject to regulatory conditions on indication, dose and labelling.

P

Pani-Flow

A specialised software system developed for collecting and analysing vaccination safety data in pandemic situations, used within the WHO/UMC pharmacovigilance infrastructure.

Periodic Safety Update Report (PSUR)

A structured, time-bound report that provides a comprehensive, worldwide review of the safety profile of a marketed medicinal product over a defined interval, integrating cumulative data and an overall safety evaluation; in ICH E2C(R2) this is harmonised as the Periodic Benefit-Risk Evaluation Report (PBRER).

Peripheral Pharmacovigilance Centre

A local or peripheral health-care facility designated within a national pharmacovigilance system as a first-line unit to detect, document and forward adverse drug reaction reports to higher-level centres.

Pharmacoepidemiology

The discipline that studies the use and effects of medicines in large populations, applying epidemiological methods to quantify patterns of use, benefits, risks and determinants of drug-related outcomes.

Pharmacology

The scientific study of the actions, mechanisms, uses and adverse effects of drugs on living organisms, encompassing pharmacokinetics and pharmacodynamics.

Pharmacovigilance

The science and activities relating to the detection, assessment, understanding and prevention of adverse effects or any other medicine-related problem.

Phytotherapy

The use of preparations derived from plants or plant parts, in a scientifically based manner, for the prevention or treatment of disease.

Placebo

An inactive preparation formulated to resemble a medicinal product but lacking active substance, used as a control in clinical trials to distinguish the effects of the investigational product from non-specific or psychological effects.

Polypharmacy

The concurrent use of multiple medicines by a patient, often defined as the regular use of several (e.g. five or more) drugs, which can increase the risk of adverse drug events and interactions.

Post-marketing

The phase after a medicinal product has been authorised and placed on the market, during which its safety and effectiveness are monitored under routine conditions of use.

Predisposing factors

Patient-related characteristics such as age, sex, genetics, comorbidities, organ impairment, concomitant medicines, alcohol use or diet that increase the likelihood of an adverse reaction or influence its clinical expression.

Pre-marketing

The development phase before a medicinal product is approved and marketed, encompassing non-clinical testing and clinical trials designed to establish its quality, safety and efficacy.[6][4]

Prescription Event Monitoring (PEM)

A form of cohort event monitoring in which prescribers are asked to report all events occurring in patients who receive a particular medicine over time, in order to characterise its safety profile in everyday clinical practice.

Prescription Only Medicine (POM)

A medicinal product that may be supplied to patients only on the order of an authorised prescriber, as defined by national medicines legislation.

Prevalence

The total number of cases of a disease or health condition in a defined population at a specified point in time (point prevalence) or over a specified period (period prevalence), expressed as a proportion of that population.

Prophylaxis

Measures, including the use of medicines or vaccines, taken to prevent the occurrence or progression of disease or other unwanted health outcomes.

R

Rational drug use

Use of medicines that is appropriate to patients' clinical needs, in doses that meet their individual requirements, for an adequate period, and at the lowest cost to them and the community.

Re-challenge

Re-administration of a medicinal product suspected of causing an adverse reaction after it has been withdrawn, to observe whether the reaction reoccurs and thereby contribute evidence to causality assessment.

Record linkage

The process of bringing together records relating to the same individual from different data sources (for example, medical records, registries or vital statistics) to enable epidemiological and pharmacovigilance analyses.

Regulatory authority

The national or regional body legally responsible for regulating medicines and related products, including their evaluation, authorisation, safety monitoring and risk-management activities (e.g. EMA, FDA, national drug regulatory agencies).

Relative risk

A measure expressing how much more (or less) likely an outcome is in an exposed group compared with an unexposed (reference) group, usually calculated as the ratio of two incidences.

Risk

The probability that a particular adverse outcome will occur in a specified population over a specified period; typically refers to the chance of harm, without directly describing its severity.

S

Serious Adverse Event or Reaction

An adverse event or adverse reaction that at any dose results in death, is life-threatening, requires inpatient hospitalisation or prolongation of existing hospitalisation, results in persistent or significant disability/incapacity, or is a congenital anomaly/birth defect; important medical events that may jeopardise the patient or require intervention to prevent such outcomes are also considered serious.

Side effect

Any unintended effect of a medicinal product that occurs at doses normally used in humans and is related to its pharmacological properties; in current regulatory usage, such effects are generally classified and reported as adverse reactions when they are harmful.

Signal

Information arising from one or multiple sources (including observations or experiments) that suggests a new potentially causal association, or a new aspect of a known association, between an intervention and an event or group of related events, judged to be of sufficient likelihood to justify verificatory action.

Spontaneous reporting

A system in which reports of suspected adverse reactions are submitted on a voluntary basis by healthcare professionals, patients or marketing authorisation holders to national pharmacovigilance centres or regulatory authorities, without a pre-defined study protocol.

Solicited Report

A safety report that originates from organised data-collection systems, such as clinical trials, non-interventional studies, registries, patient-support or named-patient programmes, or other active surveillance systems.

Suspected Unexpected Serious Adverse Drug Reaction (SUSAR)

An adverse reaction that is suspected to be related to a medicinal product, meets seriousness criteria, and whose nature or severity is not consistent with the applicable product information (e.g. Investigator's Brochure or SmPC).

T

Thalidomide

A sedative and antiemetic medicine whose use in pregnant women in the late 1950s and early 1960s caused severe congenital malformations (notably phocomelia), leading to major reforms in drug regulation and the establishment of modern pharmacovigilance; it is now restricted to specific indications under strict risk-management measures.

Traditional medicines

Knowledge, skills and practices based on theories, beliefs and experiences indigenous to different cultures, used in the maintenance of health and in the prevention, diagnosis or treatment of physical and mental illness, often involving herbal or other natural products.

U

Unexpected adverse reaction

An adverse reaction whose nature, severity or outcome is not consistent with the applicable product information (such as the SmPC or Investigator's Brochure), taking into account the characteristics of the medicinal product.

V

Vigi-Base

The global WHO database of individual case safety reports managed by the Uppsala Monitoring Centre, containing anonymised reports of suspected adverse reactions submitted by national pharmacovigilance centres participating in the WHO Programme for International Drug Monitoring.

Vigi-Flow

A web-based ICSR management system developed and maintained by the Uppsala Monitoring Centre, compliant with ICH E2B standards, that can serve as a national pharmacovigilance database and supports submission of reports to Vigi-Base.

Vigi-med

A secure communication platform for member countries of the WHO Programme for International Drug Monitoring, used to rapidly exchange information and discuss pharmacovigilance issues.

Vigi-Mine

An analytical tool within the UMC system that provides access to statistical outputs (including disproportionality measures such as the IC) for all drug–ADR combinations in Vigi-Base, supporting signal detection and exploration.

Vigi-Search

A search interface that allows authorised users to query and review individual case safety reports stored in Vigi-Base for pharmacovigilance assessment and signal evaluation.

W

WHO-ART

The WHO Adverse Reaction Terminology, an older standard terminology for coding adverse reaction information maintained by UMC, now largely superseded by MedDRA but still mapped to it for historical data.

WHO Drug Dictionary (WHO DD / WHODrug)

An international medicinal product dictionary developed within the WHO Programme for International Drug Monitoring and maintained by the Uppsala Monitoring Centre, providing structured information on medicinal products and active ingredients (including trade names, composition and other attributes) to support standardised coding and analysis in clinical trials and pharmacovigilance.

Table of Contents

CHAPTER 1

INTRODUCTION TO PHARMACOVIGILANCE

KEY OUTCOMES

Upon completion of this chapter, learners will be able to:

1. Define pharmacovigilance and articulate its comprehensive scope in healthcare systems
2. Explain the historical context and evolution of drug safety monitoring practices
3. Analyze the thalidomide tragedy and its transformative impact on pharmaceutical regulation
4. Describe the structure and function of WHO's International Drug Monitoring Programme
5. Understand the operational role of the Uppsala Monitoring Centre in global pharmacovigilance
6. Explain India's Pharmacovigilance Programme structure, objectives, and implementation
7. Identify the functions of National Coordination Centre and ADR Monitoring Centres in India

ABSTRACT

Pharmacovigilance represents a critical pillar of modern healthcare systems, dedicated to the continuous monitoring, detection, assessment, and prevention of adverse effects associated with pharmaceutical products. This chapter provides a comprehensive introduction to the science and practice of pharmacovigilance, exploring its fundamental definitions, historical evolution, and global frameworks. Beginning with the tragic thalidomide disaster that catalyzed the establishment of systematic drug safety monitoring, the chapter traces the development of international and national pharmacovigilance systems. Special emphasis is placed on the World Health Organization's International Drug Monitoring Programme, the Uppsala Monitoring Centre's pivotal role in global drug safety, and India's Pharmacovigilance Programme (PvPI) with its network of monitoring centers.

1.1. DEFINITION AND SCOPE OF PHARMACOVIGILANCE

Pharmacovigilance is the science and activities relating to the detection, assessment, understanding, and prevention of adverse effects or any other drug-related problems. The World Health Organization (WHO) defines it as the science and activities relating to the detection, assessment, understanding and prevention of adverse effects or any other medicine-related problem.

Core Objectives

The primary objectives of pharmacovigilance include improving patient care and safety, providing reliable information for risk-benefit assessment, promoting safe and rational drug use, and educating healthcare professionals and the public about medication safety. Modern pharmacovigilance extends beyond adverse drug reaction monitoring to include medication errors, quality defects, therapeutic ineffectiveness, misuse and abuse of medicines, and adverse events from counterfeit or substandard products.

Scope in Healthcare

Pharmacovigilance activities span the entire lifecycle of medicines - from preclinical development through clinical trials, regulatory approval, post-marketing surveillance, and generic drug monitoring. Special attention is given to vulnerable populations including pediatric patients, elderly individuals, pregnant women, and patients with multiple comorbidities who may not have been adequately represented in clinical trials.

1.2. HISTORY AND DEVELOPMENT OF PHARMACOVIGILANCE

The history of pharmacovigilance reflects humanity's gradual recognition that medicines, while therapeutic, can also cause harm. The evolution from isolated observations to systematic global monitoring systems represents one of the most significant developments in pharmaceutical science and public health.

Early Recognition of Drug Toxicity

Ancient civilizations recognized that certain substances could cause adverse effects. However, systematic documentation and scientific investigation of drug-related harm emerged only in the modern era. The 19th and early 20th centuries saw sporadic reports of drug toxicity, but no organized system existed for collecting, analyzing, or acting upon such information.

In 1937, the **sulfanilamide tragedy** in the United States marked an early catalyst for drug safety regulation. Over 100 deaths occurred when sulfanilamide was dissolved in diethylene glycol (a toxic solvent) and marketed as "Elixir Sulfanilamide" without adequate safety testing. This disaster led to the 1938 Federal Food, Drug, and Cosmetic Act in the US, requiring manufacturers to demonstrate drug safety before marketing.

The Thalidomide Catastrophe

The most significant turning point in pharmacovigilance history came in the late 1950s and early 1960s with the **thalidomide disaster**, which fundamentally transformed global approaches to drug safety monitoring. This tragedy demonstrated that serious adverse effects could emerge only after widespread use in populations not included in limited pre-marketing studies, particularly pregnant women.

Birth of Modern Pharmacovigilance

Following thalidomide, systematic pharmacovigilance began taking shape in the 1960s. Several countries established national adverse drug reaction monitoring systems. In 1968, the WHO launched the **International Drug Monitoring Programme**, initially involving 10 countries. This program established the foundation for global collaboration in drug safety monitoring.

The 1970s and 1980s saw refinement of pharmacovigilance methodologies, development of causality assessment tools, and expansion of national monitoring systems. Regulatory authorities began requiring post-marketing surveillance as a condition of drug approval.

The 1990s brought computerization of pharmacovigilance databases, international harmonization efforts through the International Conference on Harmonisation (ICH), and recognition of pharmacovigilance as a distinct scientific discipline. The 21st century has witnessed rapid evolution with electronic reporting systems, data mining techniques, use of social media for signal detection, and integration of pharmacogenomics into safety assessment.

1.3. THALIDOMIDE TRAGEDY AND ITS IMPACT

The thalidomide tragedy stands as the most influential event in pharmacovigilance history, fundamentally reshaping pharmaceutical regulation, drug safety monitoring, and clinical trial design worldwide.

Background and Marketing

Thalidomide was synthesized in 1953 by the German pharmaceutical company Chemie Grünenthal. Marketed from 1957 onwards under various brand names (Contergan, Distaval, Kevadon), it was promoted as a safe sedative and antiemetic, particularly for managing morning sickness in pregnant women. The drug was considered remarkably safe because it did not cause death even in large overdoses, unlike barbiturates which were commonly used sedatives at that time.

Thalidomide was sold over-the-counter in many countries without prescription requirements, reflecting the era's limited understanding of drug safety assessment. Marketing emphasized its safety profile, with some promotional materials claiming it was "completely safe" even for pregnant women and children.

The Catastrophe Unfolds

Between 1958 and 1962, approximately 10,000 children worldwide were born with severe congenital malformations, primarily **phocomelia** (severe limb deformities where hands or feet are attached close to the trunk) and other birth defects including malformations of internal organs, eyes, ears, and the cardiovascular system. The characteristic limb deformities resembled seal flippers, hence the term phocomelia from Greek words meaning "seal limb."

Dr. Widukind Lenz in Germany and Dr. William McBride in Australia independently identified the association between thalidomide use during pregnancy and congenital malformations in 1961. Their observations revealed that thalidomide was teratogenic when taken during the critical period of limb development (days 20-36 of gestation). Even brief exposure during this narrow window could cause severe birth defects.

Global Impact and Regulatory Transformation

The thalidomide disaster had profound and lasting impacts on pharmaceutical regulation and drug safety monitoring globally:

Regulatory Reforms: Countries rapidly strengthened drug approval processes. The United States enacted the Kefauver-Harris Amendment to the Food, Drug, and Cosmetic Act in 1962, requiring proof of both safety and efficacy before drug approval. Similar legislation was implemented worldwide.

Clinical Trial Requirements: The tragedy highlighted the need for adequate testing in relevant populations, proper assessment of teratogenic potential, and inclusion of reproductive toxicity studies in drug development programs.

Birth of Systematic Pharmacovigilance: Recognition that pre-marketing studies cannot detect all adverse effects, especially rare ones or those occurring in special populations, led to establishment of post-marketing surveillance systems.

International Cooperation: The tragedy demonstrated that drug safety is a global concern requiring international collaboration, directly leading to the WHO International Drug Monitoring Programme in 1968.

Lessons Learned

The thalidomide tragedy taught several enduring lessons: drugs must be assumed unsafe until proven otherwise through rigorous testing; special attention must be paid to vulnerable populations; post-marketing surveillance is essential as clinical trials have inherent limitations; and timely communication of safety concerns between countries can prevent widespread harm.

Table 1: Timeline of Thalidomide Tragedy

Year	Event
1957	Thalidomide marketed in Germany
1958-1962	Peak period of thalidomide-related birth defects
1961	Link between thalidomide and birth defects established
1961-1962	Drug withdrawn from markets worldwide
1968	WHO launches International Drug Monitoring Programme

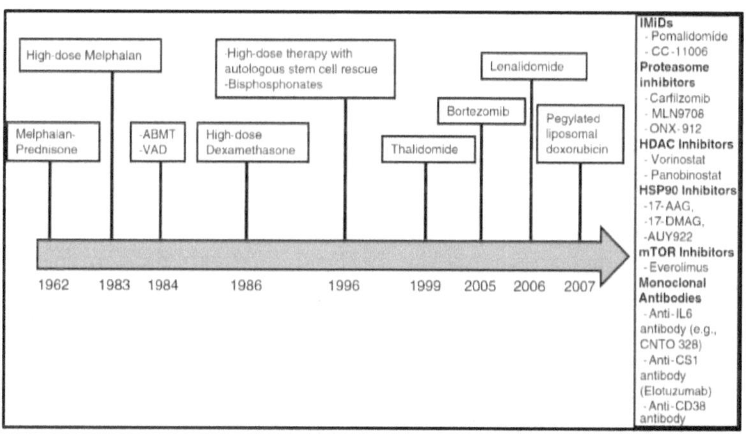

Figure 1: This timeline illustrates the critical events of the thalidomide tragedy, from initial marketing through recognition of harm and subsequent regulatory transformation.

1.4. IMPORTANCE OF SAFETY MONITORING OF MEDICINES

Continuous safety monitoring of medicines is essential for protecting public health and ensuring that the benefits of pharmaceutical therapy outweigh potential risks throughout a drug's lifecycle.

Limitations of Pre-Marketing Studies

Clinical trials conducted before drug approval have inherent limitations that necessitate ongoing post-marketing surveillance. **Sample size limitations** mean that rare adverse events (occurring in fewer than 1 in 1,000 patients) are unlikely to be detected. If a serious adverse event occurs in 1 in 10,000 patients, typical clinical trials involving hundreds to a few thousand participants would miss it entirely.

Duration of exposure in clinical trials is usually limited to weeks or months, insufficient for detecting delayed adverse effects or those requiring prolonged exposure. Chronic conditions requiring years of treatment may produce adverse effects that only manifest after extended use.

Patient selection in clinical trials excludes many real-world patients. Strict inclusion and exclusion criteria typically eliminate pregnant women, children, elderly patients, individuals with multiple comorbidities, and those taking multiple medications - precisely the populations most vulnerable to adverse effects in actual practice.

Detecting Rare and Delayed Effects

Post-marketing surveillance enables detection of **rare adverse effects** that would not appear in clinical trials of limited size. For example, serious but uncommon reactions like Stevens-Johnson syndrome, aplastic anemia, or hepatotoxicity might occur too infrequently to be observed in pre-approval studies but become apparent when millions of patients use the medicine.

Delayed effects including carcinogenicity, developmental effects on exposed children, or cumulative toxicity may only become evident years after initial exposure. Long-term safety monitoring is essential for identifying such delayed consequences.

Drug Interactions and Special Populations

Real-world medication use involves complex scenarios not adequately studied pre-marketing. **Drug-drug interactions** become apparent only when medicines are used in combination with numerous other treatments in clinical practice. **Drug-food interactions**, **drug-disease interactions**, and effects of **genetic variations** on drug metabolism and response emerge through post-marketing observation.

Public Health Protection

Effective safety monitoring protects public health by enabling early detection of safety signals, prompt regulatory action when necessary, and transparent communication of risks to healthcare providers and patients. This allows for risk minimization through updated prescribing information, restricted indications, or market withdrawal when risks outweigh benefits.

Economic Considerations

Adverse drug reactions impose substantial economic burdens through hospitalizations, prolonged hospital stays, additional treatments, disability, and lost productivity. Effective pharmacovigilance can reduce healthcare costs by preventing or minimizing adverse events through early warning systems and risk management strategies.

1.5. WHO INTERNATIONAL DRUG MONITORING PROGRAMME

The **WHO Programme for International Drug Monitoring** represents the cornerstone of global pharmacovigilance collaboration, facilitating information sharing among member countries to enhance drug safety worldwide.

Establishment and Objectives

Launched in 1968 in response to the thalidomide tragedy, the Programme initially involved 10 countries: Australia, Canada, Czechoslovakia, Federal Republic of Germany, Ireland, the Netherlands, New Zealand, Sweden, United Kingdom, and United States. Today, over 150 countries participate as full or associate members.

The primary objectives include facilitating early detection of previously unknown adverse drug reactions, identifying increases in frequency of known reactions, detecting factors that might predispose to adverse reactions, disseminating information to improve rational drug use, and promoting national pharmacovigilance development.

Structure and Function

Member countries collect adverse drug reaction reports through their national pharmacovigilance systems and submit standardized Individual Case Safety Reports (ICSRs) to the global database **VigiBase**, maintained by the Uppsala Monitoring Centre. This database contains over 25 million case reports, making it the world's largest resource of its kind.

The Programme operates through a network of **National Pharmacovigilance Centres** designated by health authorities in each member country. These centers collect, process, assess, and report adverse drug reactions according to internationally standardized formats and terminologies.

Signal Detection and Communication

WHO facilitates **signal detection** through systematic analysis of the global database, identifying potential new adverse drug reactions or changes in known reaction patterns. When signals emerge, WHO communicates findings to member states through the **WHO Pharmaceuticals Newsletter** and other channels, enabling coordinated risk assessment and regulatory action.

Capacity Building

The Programme provides technical support to developing countries for establishing and strengthening national pharmacovigilance systems. This includes training healthcare professionals, developing reporting systems, and implementing quality assurance measures.

Table 2: WHO International Drug Monitoring Programme Structure

Component	Function
Member Countries	Collect and report ADRs through national systems
National Centres	Process, assess, and submit reports to global database
Uppsala Monitoring Centre	Maintains VigiBase, conducts signal detection, provides technical support
WHO	Coordinates program, facilitates communication, promotes capacity building

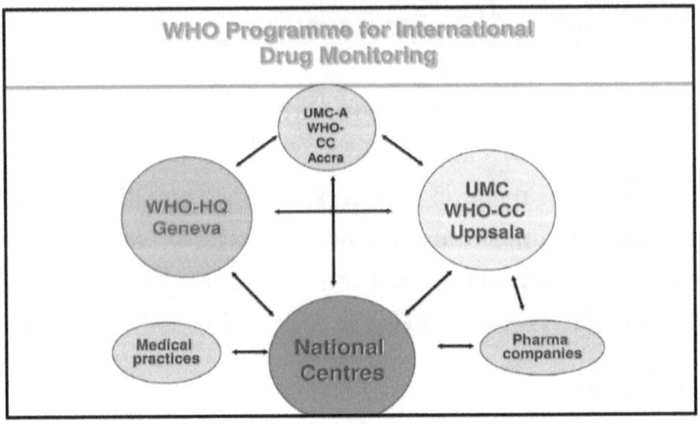

Figure 2: This organizational structure illustrates the collaborative framework of the WHO International Drug Monitoring Programme.

1.6. UPPSALA MONITORING CENTRE (UMC)

The **Uppsala Monitoring Centre** serves as the operational hub of the WHO Programme for International Drug Monitoring, providing technical and scientific leadership in global pharmacovigilance.

Background and Role

Established in 1978 and located in Uppsala, Sweden, the UMC operates under a collaborative agreement with WHO to manage the International Drug Monitoring Programme. It functions as an independent foundation, bringing together expertise in clinical pharmacology, statistics, medicine, pharmacy, and information technology.

The Centre's primary role involves maintaining and developing **VigiBase**, the WHO global database of Individual Case Safety Reports. This database receives reports from over 150 countries and serves as the foundation for international signal detection and drug safety research.

Key Functions

Database Management: UMC maintains VigiBase with rigorous quality control procedures, ensuring data standardization, consistency, and accessibility. The database includes information on suspected adverse reactions from medicines, vaccines, and other therapeutic products.

Signal Detection: UMC employs advanced statistical methods and data mining techniques for identifying safety signals. The center developed **VigiGrade**, a system for assessing the completeness and quality of case reports, and various signal detection algorithms that identify disproportionate reporting patterns suggesting potential drug safety issues.

Education and Training: UMC provides comprehensive training programs for pharmacovigilance professionals worldwide, including the highly regarded **WHO Programme** training courses that have educated thousands of professionals from member countries.

Scientific Communication: Through publications, conferences, and the **Uppsala Reports** journal, UMC disseminates pharmacovigilance knowledge and promotes best practices globally.

Tools and Resources

UMC has developed several important tools for global pharmacovigilance:

VigiBase serves as the central repository for case reports with advanced search and analysis capabilities. **VigiLyze** provides sophisticated analytical tools for signal detection and pattern recognition. **VigiFlow** offers a web-based system enabling countries to manage national databases and submit reports to VigiBase efficiently. **WHO-ART** (WHO Adverse Reaction Terminology) and support for **MedDRA** (Medical Dictionary for Regulatory Activities) provide standardized terminologies for coding adverse events.

Global Impact

UMC's work has contributed to numerous significant drug safety discoveries, including identification of previously unknown adverse reactions, characterization of rare but serious side effects, and recognition of drug safety issues requiring regulatory intervention. The Centre's collaborative approach strengthens pharmacovigilance capacity worldwide, particularly in low- and middle-income countries.

1.7. PHARMACOVIGILANCE PROGRAMME OF INDIA (PvPI)

The **Pharmacovigilance Programme of India** represents the nation's comprehensive system for monitoring the safety of medicines and ensuring patient protection through systematic adverse event detection and management.

Background and Launch

India launched the nationwide PvPI in July 2010 under the aegis of the Central Drugs Standard Control Organization (CDSCO), Ministry of Health and Family Welfare. The programme was necessitated by India's unique pharmacological landscape - serving as a major pharmaceutical manufacturing hub, having diverse genetic populations, widespread use of generic medicines, and significant consumption of both modern and traditional medicines.

The programme aims to collect reports of suspected adverse drug reactions from healthcare professionals and consumers, monitor the safety profile of medicines, generate safety signals, create awareness about drug safety, and ensure safe and rational use of medicines.

Programme Structure

PvPI operates through a hierarchical network with clearly defined roles at national, regional, and peripheral levels. The programme utilizes a multi-tier structure involving the National Coordination Centre, Zonal

Centres, Regional Centres, and peripheral ADR Monitoring Centres (AMCs) located in hospitals across India.

Operational Framework

The programme functions through **spontaneous reporting** where healthcare professionals and patients report suspected adverse drug reactions voluntarily. Reports are collected using standardized forms and submitted either online through the PvPI portal or offline through designated channels.

Each report undergoes systematic evaluation including causality assessment to determine the likelihood that the drug caused the reported reaction, severity assessment, and predictability determination. Reports meeting quality criteria are forwarded to VigiBase, contributing to international drug safety knowledge.

Achievements and Expansion

Since its inception, PvPI has achieved significant milestones including establishment of over 300 ADR Monitoring Centres across India, collection of hundreds of thousands of adverse drug reaction reports, integration with international databases through WHO Programme membership, and generation of important safety signals leading to regulatory actions.

The programme conducts regular training and awareness activities for healthcare professionals, develops educational materials, and promotes a culture of safety reporting across Indian healthcare institutions.

Challenges and Future Directions

PvPI faces challenges common to pharmacovigilance systems in large, diverse countries including underreporting of adverse events, need for greater awareness among healthcare professionals, ensuring report quality and completeness, and coverage expansion to remote areas. Future directions include strengthening existing monitoring centers, incorporating technology solutions for efficient reporting, enhancing consumer reporting mechanisms, and integrating pharmacovigilance into routine healthcare practice.

1.8. NATIONAL COORDINATION CENTRE (NCC)

The **National Coordination Centre** functions as the apex body of India's Pharmacovigilance Programme, providing strategic direction, technical oversight, and operational coordination for the entire national network.

Location and Administrative Structure

The NCC is located at the **Indian Pharmacopoeia Commission** (IPC) in Ghaziabad, Uttar Pradesh. Operating under the Ministry of Health and Family Welfare and CDSCO oversight, the NCC serves as India's designated WHO collaborating centre for pharmacovigilance in public health programmes.

Core Responsibilities

The NCC fulfills multiple critical functions within the national pharmacovigilance framework. **Programme coordination** involves overall management and monitoring of PvPI activities nationwide, ensuring standardized implementation across all monitoring centers, and maintaining communication with CDSCO for regulatory coordination.

Data management represents a major responsibility, with the NCC maintaining the national pharmacovigilance database, ensuring data quality through validation procedures, analyzing adverse drug reaction reports for signal detection, and submitting reports to VigiBase as per WHO requirements.

Training and capacity building activities include developing training modules and educational materials, conducting regular workshops for healthcare professionals, organizing conferences and seminars on pharmacovigilance, and providing technical guidance to monitoring centers.

Communication and dissemination involves publishing safety alerts and newsletters, maintaining the PvPI portal with information resources, communicating with stakeholders including healthcare professionals and patients, and coordinating with regulatory authorities for necessary actions.

Technical Functions

The NCC performs **causality assessment** using standardized algorithms to determine the relationship between drugs and reported adverse events. **Signal detection and evaluation** employs statistical methods to identify potential new adverse drug reactions or changes in known reaction patterns.

Regulatory support includes providing technical inputs to CDSCO for regulatory decisions, contributing to risk-benefit assessments of medicines, participating in expert committee deliberations on drug safety, and supporting labeling changes or regulatory actions based on safety data.

International Collaboration

As India's representative to the WHO Programme for International Drug Monitoring, the NCC facilitates information exchange with international pharmacovigilance community, participates in global signal detection activities, adopts international best practices, and contributes Indian safety data to global knowledge.

Table 3: PvPI Organizational Structure

Level	Component	Primary Function
National	National Coordination Centre (NCC) - IPC Ghaziabad	Overall coordination, database management, signal detection
Regional	Zonal and Regional Centres (5 zones)	Regional coordination, training, quality oversight
Peripheral	ADR Monitoring Centres (AMCs) - 300+ hospitals	Direct collection of ADR reports from healthcare professionals
Reporting	Healthcare professionals and patients	Report suspected adverse drug reactions

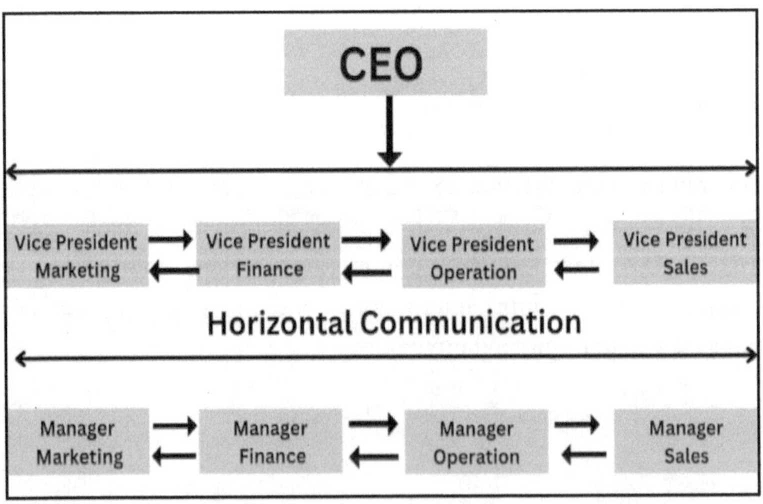

Figure 3: The PvPI operates through a hierarchical structure with information flowing upward from individual reporters through monitoring centers to regional coordination and ultimately to the National Coordination Centre.

1.9. ADR MONITORING CENTRES (AMCs) IN INDIA

ADR Monitoring Centres form the foundational network of India's Pharmacovigilance Programme, serving as primary collection points for adverse drug reaction reports across the country's diverse healthcare landscape.

Establishment and Distribution

AMCs are established in various healthcare institutions including government medical colleges, large government hospitals, and private tertiary care hospitals. The selection criteria for AMC designation include availability of qualified healthcare professionals, adequate patient load ensuring sufficient exposure to diverse medications, institutional commitment to pharmacovigilance activities, and infrastructure for report collection and processing.

Currently, over 300 AMCs operate across India, strategically distributed to ensure geographical coverage including urban, semi-urban, and rural areas. Each state typically has multiple AMCs proportionate to population and healthcare infrastructure.

Functions and Responsibilities

Report collection constitutes the primary function, where AMCs receive adverse drug reaction reports from healthcare professionals including physicians, pharmacists, nurses, and other clinical staff. Patient and consumer reports are increasingly encouraged and facilitated through accessible reporting mechanisms.

Initial assessment involves reviewing reports for completeness, conducting causality assessment using standardized algorithms, assessing severity and seriousness of reactions, and documenting relevant clinical information and outcomes.

Documentation and reporting requires maintaining records of all collected reports, entering data into the national pharmacovigilance database through the PvPI portal, and forwarding reports to regional centers and ultimately to the National Coordination Centre.

Awareness and training activities include conducting educational sessions for hospital staff, organizing continuing medical education programs on pharmacovigilance, creating awareness among patients about reporting adverse effects, and promoting a reporting culture within the institution.

Operational Framework

Each AMC designates a **nodal officer**, typically a faculty member or senior clinician with training in pharmacovigilance, responsible for overall coordination. A **pharmacovigilance team** including pharmacists, clinical pharmacologists, and support staff assists in data collection and processing.

AMCs utilize standardized reporting forms aligned with international formats, ensuring consistency and compatibility with global databases. Both online reporting through the PvPI web portal and offline reporting via paper forms or email are accommodated.

Challenges Faced by AMCs

Despite progress, AMCs encounter several operational challenges. **Underreporting** remains a significant issue, with many adverse reactions going unreported due to time constraints, lack of awareness, fear of legal implications, or perception that only serious reactions need reporting.

Resource limitations including insufficient staff dedicated to pharmacovigilance, competing clinical responsibilities, and inadequate infrastructure in some centers affect operational efficiency. **Training needs** remain substantial, requiring continuous education to maintain pharmacovigilance competency among rotating staff and growing networks.

Best Practices and Success Factors

Successful AMCs demonstrate certain common characteristics: strong institutional commitment reflected in dedicated resources and administrative support; integration of pharmacovigilance into routine clinical practice; regular training and motivation of reporting healthcare professionals; efficient communication channels between reporters and pharmacovigilance teams; and systematic follow-up of reported cases to obtain complete information and outcomes.

The expansion and strengthening of the AMC network represents a critical priority for enhancing India's pharmacovigilance capabilities, ensuring comprehensive medication safety monitoring across the nation's diverse population and healthcare settings.

Pharmacovigilance has evolved from reactive responses to drug disasters into a proactive, systematic science essential for public health protection. The thalidomide tragedy demonstrated the critical need for continuous safety monitoring beyond pre-marketing clinical trials, catalyzing establishment of national and international pharmacovigilance systems. The WHO International Drug Monitoring Programme, supported by the Uppsala Monitoring Centre, provides the global framework for collaborative drug safety surveillance, while national programs like India's PvPI implement systematic monitoring adapted to local contexts.

The comprehensive infrastructure spanning from individual ADR Monitoring Centres through regional coordination to national and international levels enables detection of rare adverse effects, identification of risk factors, and implementation of risk minimization measures. As pharmacovigilance continues evolving with technological advances and expanding scope, its fundamental purpose remains unchanged: ensuring that medicines benefit patients while minimizing preventable harm. The success of pharmacovigilance systems depends ultimately on active participation by healthcare professionals, regulatory authorities, pharmaceutical industry, and patients working collaboratively toward the shared goal of medication safety.

Best Practices and Success Factors

Successful AMCs demonstrate certain common characteristics: strong institutional commitment reflected in dedicated resources and administrative support; integration of pharmacovigilance into routine clinical practice; regular training and motivation of reporting healthcare professionals; efficient communication channels between reporters and pharmacovigilance teams; and systematic follow-up of reported cases to obtain complete information and outcomes.

Pharmacovigilance has transformed dramatically from reactive responses to drug crises into a proactive science safeguarding public health, with the thalidomide tragedy serving as a pivotal wake-up call that pre-marketing trials alone fall short, spurring the birth of national and international monitoring systems. Globally, the WHO's International Drug Monitoring Programme, anchored by the Uppsala Monitoring Centre, enables collaborative vigilance, while India's PvPI adapts this framework to local realities through a robust network of ADR Monitoring Centres, regional coordinators, national hubs, and international ties - masterfully detecting rare adverse effects, identifying risks, and enacting minimization strategies. As technological advances and an expanding scope propel it forward, pharmacovigilance's enduring mission remains clear: ensuring medicines heal without needless harm. Ultimately, its success rests on the united efforts of healthcare professionals, regulators, the pharmaceutical industry, and patients in pursuit of safer therapy.

CHAPTER 2

INTRODUCTION TO ADVERSE DRUG REACTIONS (ADRs)

KEY OUTCOMES

Upon completion of this chapter, learners will be able to:

1. Define adverse drug reactions using internationally standardized terminology
2. Differentiate between various types of adverse medication events
3. Apply multiple classification systems for categorizing ADRs
4. Explain the Rawlins and Thompson classification of Type A and Type B reactions
5. Describe the DoTS classification system and its clinical applications
6. Perform causality assessment using WHO-UMC scale and Naranjo Algorithm
7. Assess severity and seriousness of adverse drug reactions according to regulatory criteria
8. Evaluate predictability and preventability of ADRs
9. Implement appropriate management strategies for adverse drug reactions
10. Appreciate the economic burden of ADRs on healthcare systems

ABSTRACT

Adverse Drug Reactions (ADRs) represent a significant healthcare challenge, contributing to morbidity, mortality, and substantial economic burden globally. This chapter provides comprehensive coverage of ADR fundamentals, exploring precise definitions, classification systems, detection methodologies, and management strategies. Beginning with standardized terminology, the chapter examines multiple classification frameworks including the traditional Rawlins and Thompson system distinguishing Type A and Type B reactions, and the more contemporary DoTS classification incorporating Dose-relatedness, Timing, and Susceptibility factors. Detailed exploration of causality assessment methodologies, particularly the WHO-UMC scale and Naranjo Algorithm, equips learners with practical tools for determining drug-reaction relationships. The chapter addresses severity grading, seriousness criteria, predictability, and preventability assessments essential for clinical decision-making and regulatory reporting. Management principles for ADRs and analysis of their economic impact complete this foundational understanding necessary for effective pharmacovigilance practice.

2.1. DEFINITIONS

Precise terminology forms the foundation of effective pharmacovigilance communication and practice. International harmonization of definitions ensures consistency in reporting, assessment, and regulatory decision-making across borders.

Adverse Drug Reaction (ADR)

The World Health Organization defines an adverse drug reaction as "a response to a drug which is noxious and unintended, and which occurs at doses normally used in man for the prophylaxis, diagnosis, or therapy of disease, or for the modification of physiological function." This definition emphasizes several critical elements.

First, the response must be noxious (harmful or undesirable), distinguishing ADRs from therapeutic effects or benign reactions. Second, it must be unintended, occurring outside the desired therapeutic outcome. Third, it occurs at normal therapeutic doses, differentiating ADRs from effects of overdose or poisoning. Fourth, the definition encompasses drugs used for any medical purpose including prevention, diagnosis, treatment, or physiological modification.

This classical WHO definition applies to reactions occurring from established, approved uses of medicines. It excludes effects from intentional or accidental overdose, medication errors (though these may lead to ADRs), and therapeutic failures.

Adverse Event (AE)

An adverse event represents a broader concept defined as "any untoward medical occurrence in a patient or clinical trial subject administered a pharmaceutical product, which does not necessarily have a causal relationship with the treatment." This definition is particularly important in clinical trial contexts.

The key distinction from ADR lies in causality—an adverse event need not be causally related to the drug, merely temporally associated. Any negative health occurrence during drug therapy qualifies as an adverse event, whether caused by the drug, underlying disease, concurrent conditions, or coincidental factors.

Side Effect

A side effect refers to any unintended effect of a pharmaceutical product occurring at normal doses, which may be beneficial, neutral, or harmful. Not all side effects are adverse—some may be therapeutically exploited or clinically insignificant. For example, drowsiness from antihistamines might be adverse in some contexts but therapeutically useful when managing insomnia.

Serious Adverse Event/Reaction

A serious adverse event or reaction meets specific regulatory criteria defined consistently across major regulatory authorities. An event is considered serious if it results in death, is life-threatening, requires inpatient hospitalization or prolongation of existing hospitalization, results in persistent or significant disability or incapacity, is a congenital anomaly or birth defect, or is a medically important event requiring intervention to prevent one of the other serious outcomes.

The term "life-threatening" refers to events where the patient was at immediate risk of death at the time of the event, not reactions that hypothetically might cause death if more severe.

Unexpected Adverse Reaction

An unexpected adverse reaction is one whose nature, severity, or outcome is not consistent with the reference safety information for the product. For marketed medicines, the reference safety information is typically the approved product labeling. In clinical trials, it refers to the investigator's brochure or protocol safety information.

Unexpectedness relates to whether the specific reaction is documented in available product information, not merely whether it is theoretically possible. A known reaction occurring with greater severity than previously documented may also be considered unexpected.

2.2. CLASSIFICATION OF ADRs

Classification systems for adverse drug reactions serve multiple purposes: facilitating understanding of underlying mechanisms, guiding clinical management, predicting potential reactions, and organizing pharmacovigilance data systematically. Multiple classification frameworks exist, each offering unique perspectives on ADR characteristics.

Basic Classifications

ADRs can be classified by various criteria. Severity ranges from mild (requiring minimal or no intervention) through moderate (requiring intervention but not life-threatening) to severe (life-threatening, causing permanent damage, or resulting in death).

Onset timing distinguishes acute reactions (occurring within hours), subacute reactions (days to weeks), and chronic or latent reactions (months to years). Organ system affected provides anatomical classification including dermatological, hematological, hepatic, renal, cardiovascular, and neurological reactions.

Relationship to dose separates dose-dependent reactions (increasing in frequency or severity with higher doses) from dose-independent reactions (occurring unpredictably regardless of dose).

2.3. RAWLINS AND THOMPSON CLASSIFICATION

The Rawlins and Thompson classification, introduced in 1977, remains one of the most widely used ADR classification systems, distinguishing reactions based on their relationship to known pharmacology and predictability.

Type A Reactions (Augmented)

Type A reactions represent augmented or exaggerated pharmacological effects of the drug occurring at therapeutic doses. These reactions are extensions of the drug's known pharmacological actions and constitute approximately 80% of all ADRs.

Characteristics include dose-dependency (increasing frequency and severity with higher doses), predictability based on drug pharmacology, common occurrence (relatively high incidence), typically reversibility upon dose reduction or drug discontinuation, and generally low mortality despite potentially significant morbidity.

Examples include bleeding with anticoagulants, hypoglycemia with insulin or oral hypoglycemic agents, bradycardia with beta-blockers, constipation with opioids, and sedation with benzodiazepines. These reactions relate directly to the therapeutic mechanism - anticoagulants prevent clotting (therapeutic) but can cause bleeding (adverse); hypoglycemics lower blood sugar (therapeutic) but can cause excessive reduction (adverse).

Management typically involves dose adjustment, careful monitoring of patients at higher risk, use of minimum effective doses, and consideration of individual patient factors affecting drug response such as age, renal or hepatic function, and concurrent medications.

Type B Reactions (Bizarre)

Type B reactions are bizarre, idiosyncratic reactions unrelated to the drug's known pharmacological actions. These reactions are typically immunological or have genetic predisposition, constituting approximately 20% of ADRs but causing disproportionate morbidity and mortality.

Characteristics include dose-independence (occurring unpredictably regardless of dose), unpredictability (not based on known pharmacology), rarity (low incidence), often high severity and mortality, and mechanism involving immunological reactions or genetic variations in drug metabolism.

Examples include anaphylaxis to penicillin, Stevens-Johnson syndrome with various drugs, malignant hyperthermia with anesthetics, aplastic anemia with chloramphenicol, and hemolytic anemia in G6PD deficiency patients taking certain drugs.

Management requires immediate drug discontinuation, avoidance of the drug and often structurally related compounds in future, symptomatic and supportive treatment, and documentation to prevent re-exposure.

Additional Types

Some authorities have expanded the original classification to include additional categories:

Type C Reactions (Chronic) relate to long-term drug use, such as opioid dependence or tardive dyskinesia from antipsychotics.

Type D Reactions (Delayed) manifest significantly after drug exposure, including carcinogenesis or teratogenesis.

Type E Reactions (End-of-use) occur upon drug withdrawal, such as adrenal insufficiency after corticosteroid withdrawal.

Type F Reactions (Failure) involve unexpected therapeutic failure, often due to drug interactions or genetic variations affecting drug metabolism.

2.4. DoTS CLASSIFICATION

The DoTS classification system (Dose-relatedness, Timing, and Susceptibility), proposed by Aronson and Ferner in 2003, represents a more comprehensive, multidimensional approach to ADR classification that addresses limitations of the traditional Type A / Type B system.

Conceptual Framework

DoTS recognizes that adverse drug reactions are complex phenomena requiring consideration of multiple factors simultaneously. Rather than forcing reactions into discrete categories, DoTS characterizes each ADR along three independent axes: dose-relatedness, timing of reaction, and patient susceptibility factors.

Dose-Relatedness (D)

This dimension examines the relationship between drug dose and occurrence or severity of the adverse reaction. Toxic reactions occur at supratherapeutic doses in most patients, typically showing clear dose-response relationships. Examples include paracetamol hepatotoxicity and digoxin toxicity.

Collateral reactions occur at standard therapeutic doses and represent effects related to the drug's pharmacological actions but distinct from the primary therapeutic effect. Most Type A reactions fall into this category, such as beta-blocker-induced bronchospasm or anticholinergic effects of antihistamines.

Hypersusceptibility reactions occur at subtherapeutic doses in susceptible individuals due to pharmacokinetic or pharmacodynamic variations. Examples include severe reactions in patients with genetic polymorphisms affecting drug metabolism or increased receptor sensitivity.

Timing (T)

The temporal relationship between drug administration and reaction onset provides important mechanistic and diagnostic information. Time-independent reactions can occur at any time during drug therapy without clear temporal patterns, such as unpredictable immunological reactions.

Time-dependent reactions follow characteristic temporal patterns. First-dose reactions occur with initial administration, commonly seen with immunological phenomena like anaphylaxis or pharmacological effects like first-dose hypotension with alpha-blockers.

Early reactions appear early in treatment but not necessarily with the first dose, such as nausea with many drugs where tolerance may develop. Intermediate reactions emerge after days to weeks of treatment, exemplified by drug-induced rashes or photosensitivity.

Late reactions manifest after prolonged exposure, including tardive dyskinesia from antipsychotics or osteoporosis from corticosteroids. Delayed reactions occur significantly after drug discontinuation, such as vaginal adenocarcinoma in daughters of women who took diethylstilbestrol during pregnancy.

Susceptibility (S)

Patient-specific factors that increase vulnerability to adverse reactions encompass genetic, pathological, demographic, and environmental variables. Genetic susceptibility includes polymorphisms in drug-metabolizing enzymes (cytochrome P450 variants), receptor variations affecting drug response, and conditions like glucose-6-phosphate dehydrogenase deficiency predisposing to hemolysis.

Age-related susceptibility reflects pharmacokinetic and pharmacodynamic changes. Pediatric patients may lack mature enzyme systems, while elderly patients often have reduced renal clearance and altered drug distribution. Sex differences affect susceptibility through hormonal influences, body composition variations, and sex-linked genetic factors.

Hepatic or renal disease reduces drug elimination, increasing exposure and toxicity risk. Drug interactions involving pharmacokinetic (affecting drug levels) or pharmacodynamic (affecting drug effects) mechanisms increase reaction susceptibility.

Disease states may predispose to specific reactions; for example, heart failure patients are more susceptible to fluid retention from NSAIDs, and patients with Parkinson's disease are vulnerable to extrapyramidal effects from antipsychotics.

Clinical Application

DoTS classification enables more precise characterization of adverse reactions than dichotomous Type A/Type B systems. A single reaction is described across all three dimensions, providing comprehensive understanding useful for predicting risk, identifying vulnerable patients, implementing preventive measures, and understanding mechanisms.

For example, statin-induced myopathy would be characterized as: dose-related (collateral effect at therapeutic doses, more common with higher doses), timing (intermediate to late reaction after weeks to months), and susceptibility (increased risk with genetic variations in drug transporters, concurrent use of CYP3A4 inhibitors, hypothyroidism, or renal impairment).

2.5. DETECTION AND REPORTING OF ADRs

Early detection and comprehensive reporting of adverse drug reactions form the foundation of effective pharmacovigilance, enabling signal generation, risk assessment, and protective regulatory actions.

Detection Methods

Spontaneous reporting remains the cornerstone of ADR detection worldwide. Healthcare professionals and increasingly patients voluntarily report suspected adverse reactions to national pharmacovigilance authorities. While simple and cost-effective, spontaneous reporting suffers from significant underreporting, with estimates suggesting only 1-10% of serious ADRs are reported.

Intensive monitoring involves systematic, active surveillance in specific settings such as hospital wards or clinics, using dedicated personnel to identify and document all adverse events. This approach yields higher detection rates but requires substantial resources.

Prescription event monitoring follows cohorts of patients prescribed specific medicines, recording all events without initial judgment of causality. This method provides denominator data (number of patients exposed) enabling incidence calculation.

Electronic health record surveillance increasingly utilizes automated algorithms to screen electronic medical records for potential ADRs based on predefined criteria, laboratory abnormalities, or characteristic symptom patterns. This technology-enabled approach offers efficiency and comprehensiveness but requires sophisticated systems and validation.

Who Should Report?

All healthcare professionals including physicians, dentists, pharmacists, nurses, and allied health workers have professional and ethical obligations to report suspected ADRs, particularly serious or unexpected reactions. Patient and consumer reporting has gained recognition as a valuable complementary source, often providing unique perspectives on symptom impact and chronology not captured in clinical records.

Pharmaceutical manufacturers have legal obligations to report adverse events that come to their attention through various channels including clinical trials, spontaneous reports, scientific literature, and regulatory inquiries.

What Should Be Reported?

Priority for reporting includes all serious or unexpected adverse reactions, even if causality is uncertain; reactions to new medicines (typically those marketed less than five years); suspected interactions between medicines; reactions resulting from medication errors; suspected adverse effects from excipients; suspected lack of efficacy particularly of life-saving medications; and suspected transmission of infectious agents through medicines.

The principle is "when in doubt, report" - causality assessment is performed systematically by pharmacovigilance experts, and healthcare professionals should report suspected reactions even without certainty of causal relationship.

Reporting Mechanisms

Most countries provide multiple reporting channels to facilitate accessibility. Online portals offer web-based forms with structured fields ensuring completeness and immediate data capture. Paper-based reporting using standardized forms remains available, particularly in resource-limited settings. Telephone reporting to pharmacovigilance centers enables immediate consultation and assistance. Mobile applications increasingly provide convenient reporting interfaces for healthcare professionals and patients.

Essential Information

Quality ADR reports contain several critical elements: identifiable patient (initials, age, sex, unique identifier), identifiable reporter (for follow-up communication), suspected medicine(s) (name, dose, route, dates of administration), suspected reaction (description, onset date, outcome), and relevant clinical information (indication for drug use, concomitant medications, underlying conditions).

Follow-up information may be sought to complete initial reports, including outcome of reaction, dechallenge and rechallenge information, laboratory results, and additional clinical details supporting causality assessment.

2.6. METHODS IN CAUSALITY ASSESSMENT

Causality assessment represents the systematic evaluation of the likelihood that a particular medicine caused an observed adverse event. This process is fundamental to pharmacovigilance, distinguishing true adverse drug reactions from coincidental associations.

Principles of Causality

Establishing causality involves evaluating several key elements. Temporal relationship requires that drug administration precede the adverse event with biologically plausible timing. Biological plausibility considers whether the reaction is consistent with known pharmacology or previous knowledge about the drug or class.

Dechallenge evaluates whether reaction resolution or improvement follows drug discontinuation, supporting (though not proving) causality. Rechallenge provides the strongest evidence when reaction recurs upon intentional or inadvertent re-exposure, though rechallenge is rarely performed for ethical and safety reasons, particularly with serious reactions.

Alternative explanations must be considered - concurrent diseases, other medications, or environmental factors might explain the observed event. Previous knowledge about similar reactions with the drug or related compounds influences causality likelihood.

Challenges in Assessment

Several factors complicate causality assessment. Polypharmacy is common in clinical practice, making attribution to a specific drug difficult when patients take multiple medications. Underlying diseases may produce symptoms similar to potential adverse reactions. Time-dependent patterns vary widely-some reactions occur immediately while others emerge after prolonged exposure or even following discontinuation.

Rare reactions lack extensive prior documentation, making biological plausibility assessment difficult. Confounding factors including age, genetics, diet, and concurrent exposures influence both drug response and disease progression.

Standardized Assessment Methods

Multiple standardized algorithms have been developed to improve consistency and reproducibility of causality assessment. These tools typically assign probability categories based on systematic evaluation of relevant factors.

2.7. WHO-UMC CAUSALITY ASSESSMENT SCALE

The WHO-UMC Causality Assessment Scale represents a globally recognized, practical system for standardizing causality evaluation in pharmacovigilance, used extensively by national pharmacovigilance centers worldwide.

Categories and Criteria

The system classifies adverse event causality into six categories based on clinical-pharmacological criteria:

Certain: A clinical event occurring in a plausible temporal relationship to drug administration that cannot be explained by concurrent disease or other drugs or chemicals. The response to withdrawal (dechallenge) should be clinically plausible. The event must be definitive pharmacologically or phenomenologically, using satisfactory rechallenge procedure if necessary. This highest certainty level is rarely achieved in clinical practice due to ethical constraints on rechallenge and presence of multiple potential causes.

Probable/Likely: A clinical event with reasonable temporal relationship to drug administration, unlikely to be attributed to concurrent disease or other drugs or chemicals, and with reasonable response to withdrawal. Rechallenge information is not required. This category applies when the reaction is known for the drug, timing is appropriate, alternative causes are less likely, and improvement follows drug cessation.

Possible: A clinical event with reasonable temporal relationship to drug administration but that could also be explained by concurrent disease or other drugs or chemicals. Information on drug withdrawal may be lacking or unclear. This category encompasses many spontaneous reports where multiple potential causes exist and complete information is unavailable.

Unlikely: A clinical event with temporal relationship to drug administration that makes causal relationship improbable, and in which other drugs, chemicals, or underlying disease provide plausible explanations. This applies when alternative causes clearly better explain the event or timing is inappropriate for drug causation.

Conditional/Unclassified: A clinical event reported as an adverse reaction where more data for proper assessment is needed, or additional data is under examination. This interim category applies during information gathering or pending expert review.

Unassessable/Unclassifiable: A report suggesting an adverse reaction that cannot be judged because information is insufficient or contradictory, and cannot be supplemented or verified. Many spontaneous reports fall into this category due to incomplete information despite follow-up efforts.

Application Process

Assessment begins with verifying temporal relationship - whether drug administration preceded the event with appropriate timing. Next, evaluating whether known or expected reaction for the drug class increases likelihood. Alternative explanations including concomitant medications, underlying or concurrent diseases, and other environmental factors are systematically considered.

Dechallenge information - whether reaction resolved or improved upon drug discontinuation - is evaluated if available. Rechallenge data, though rarely available, provides strongest evidence. All evidence is weighed collectively to assign the most appropriate category.

Strengths and Limitations

The WHO-UMC scale's strengths include global acceptance and standardization, relative simplicity enabling widespread use, and sufficient flexibility for diverse clinical scenarios. However, limitations include subjectivity in applying criteria, dependence on information completeness, inability to provide quantitative probability, and variability in assessment between evaluators.

Table 4: WHO-UMC Causality Assessment Process

Assessment Step	Key Questions	Evidence Evaluated
Temporal Relationship	Did drug precede event with appropriate timing?	Administration dates, reaction onset
Known Reaction	Is this reaction documented for the drug?	Product information, literature
Alternative Causes	Could other factors explain the event?	Concomitant drugs, diseases, exposures
Dechallenge	Did reaction improve after stopping drug?	Clinical course after discontinuation
Rechallenge	Did reaction recur on re-exposure?	Response to re-administration (rarely available)

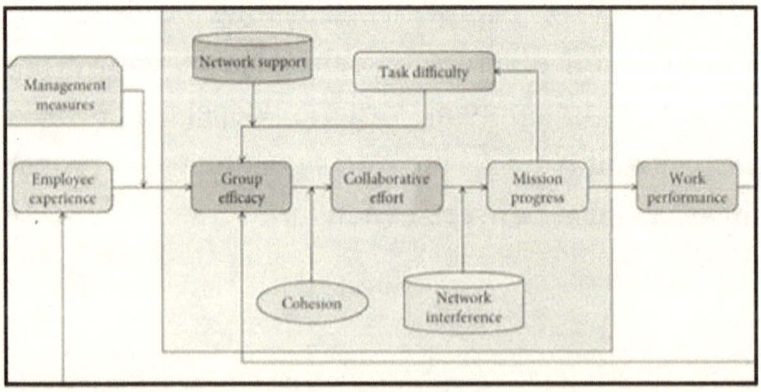

Figure. 4: This flowchart illustrates the systematic process of causality assessment using the WHO-UMC scale. Each step evaluates specific aspects of the drug-event relationship, with evidence accumulated across all dimensions informing the final causality category assignment.

2.8 NARANJO ALGORITHM

The Naranjo Adverse Drug Reaction Probability Scale, developed by Naranjo and colleagues in 1981, provides a quantitative, standardized method for causality assessment using a scoring system based on ten weighted questions.

Structure and Scoring

The algorithm consists of ten questions, each answered as "Yes," "No," or "Do not know/Not applicable." Each answer receives a predetermined score (positive, negative, or zero), and total scores are summed to assign probability categories.

Question 1: Are there previous conclusive reports on this reaction? (Yes +1, No 0, Unknown 0) This evaluates whether the reaction is documented in literature or product information.

Question 2: Did the adverse event appear after the suspected drug was administered? (Yes +2, No -1, Unknown 0) This fundamental question establishes temporal relationship.

Question 3: Did the adverse reaction improve when the drug was discontinued or a specific antagonist was administered? (Yes +1, No 0, Unknown 0) This assesses dechallenge response.

Question 4: Did the adverse reaction reappear when the drug was readministered? (Yes +2, No -1, Unknown 0) Rechallenge provides strong evidence but is rarely performed.

Question 5: Are there alternative causes that could have caused the reaction? (Yes -1, No +2, Unknown 0) This evaluates competing explanations including concurrent diseases or medications.

Question 6: Did the reaction reappear when a placebo was given? (Yes -1, No +1, Unknown 0) This question is rarely applicable outside clinical trial settings.

Question 7: Was the drug detected in blood or other fluids in concentrations known to be toxic? (Yes +1, No 0, Unknown 0) This applies when therapeutic drug monitoring or toxicology data is available.

Question 8: Was the reaction more severe when the dose was increased, or less severe when the dose was decreased? (Yes +1, No 0, Unknown 0) This evaluates dose-response relationship.

Question 9: Did the patient have a similar reaction to the same or similar drugs in any previous exposure? (Yes +1, No 0, Unknown 0) Previous personal history increases likelihood.

Question 10: Was the adverse event confirmed by any objective evidence? (Yes +1, No 0, Unknown 0) This values laboratory, radiological, or other objective confirmation.

Score Interpretation

Total scores are categorized as follows: Definite (score ≥ 9) indicates very high probability of drug causation; Probable (score 5-8) suggests likely drug causation; Possible (score 1-4) indicates causation is plausible but uncertain; Doubtful (score ≤ 0) suggests drug is unlikely cause.

Practical Application

The Naranjo Algorithm is applied retrospectively to individual case reports. Each question is answered systematically based on available clinical information, scores are summed, and the total determines probability category. The structured approach reduces subjectivity and improves reproducibility compared to unstructured clinical judgment.

Advantages and Limitations

Advantages include quantitative scoring enabling comparison across cases, relative objectivity through standardized questions, good inter-rater reliability, and wide acceptance in clinical research. Limitations include equal weighting of questions despite varying clinical importance, inability to capture all relevant clinical nuances, dependence on information availability, and lower discriminatory power for scores in the middle range.

2.9 SEVERITY AND SERIOUSNESS ASSESSMENT

Proper assessment of ADR severity and seriousness is crucial for determining appropriate management, reporting requirements, and regulatory priorities. These two concepts, while related, have distinct definitions and implications.

Severity Assessment

Severity refers to the intensity of the adverse reaction and its impact on patient function and well-being. Severity is typically graded on a three or four-point scale:

Mild: The reaction is usually transient, requires no specific treatment or intervention, does not significantly interfere with patient's usual activities, and causes minimal discomfort. Examples include mild nausea, slight headache, or minor skin rash.

Moderate: The reaction causes some interference with usual activities, may require some therapeutic intervention, produces discomfort but is not life-threatening or permanently disabling, and may warrant drug dose adjustment. Examples include moderate nausea requiring antiemetics, significant but not severe rash, or mild elevation of liver enzymes.

Severe: The reaction significantly interferes with patient's usual activities, requires intensive therapeutic intervention, is potentially life-threatening or permanently disabling, usually necessitates drug discontinuation or hospitalization, and may result in persistent or significant disability. Examples include severe hepatotoxicity, anaphylaxis, or Stevens-Johnson syndrome.

Some grading systems add a fourth category, life-threatening, for reactions placing patient at immediate risk of death.

Seriousness Criteria

Seriousness is a regulatory definition based on specific outcome criteria rather than symptom intensity. An adverse event is classified as serious if it meets any of the following criteria:

Results in death: The event directly or indirectly led to patient death. Causality assessment determines whether the drug contributed to death.

Is life-threatening: The patient was at immediate risk of death at the time of the event. This refers to actual risk at the time, not potential risk if the reaction had been more severe.

Requires inpatient hospitalization or prolongation of existing hospitalization: The event necessitates admission to hospital or extends an existing hospital stay. Hospitalization solely for convenience, social reasons, or elective procedures generally does not qualify.

Results in persistent or significant disability/incapacity: The event causes substantial disruption of person's ability to conduct normal life functions. This includes both physical and psychological disabilities.

Is a congenital anomaly/birth defect: Suspected adverse effects on offspring exposed in utero qualify as serious regardless of other criteria.

Is a medically important event: Events that may not meet other criteria but represent significant medical hazards requiring intervention to prevent serious outcomes are classified as serious based on medical judgment. Examples include development of drug dependence, seizures not resulting in hospitalization, or blood dyscrasias.

Relationship Between Severity and Seriousness

Severity and seriousness, though related, are distinct concepts. A reaction can be severe but not serious (e.g., intense but transient headache managed at home), or serious but not severe (e.g., hospitalization for observation after suspected anaphylaxis that resolved before hospital arrival, or mild congenital anomaly). However, many serious reactions are also severe, and severity influences medical importance assessment.

Reporting requirements typically prioritize serious reactions for regulatory notification, while severity assessment guides clinical management decisions. Both parameters are important in pharmacovigilance assessment and should be documented for all ADR reports.

2.10 PREDICTABILITY AND PREVENTABILITY ASSESSMENT

Assessment of whether adverse reactions were predictable and preventable provides valuable insights for improving medication safety and guiding risk management strategies.

Predictability Assessment

Predictability refers to whether an adverse reaction could be anticipated based on available information about the drug's pharmacology, previous clinical experience, patient characteristics, or known risk factors.

Predictable (Type A) reactions: These can be anticipated based on the drug's pharmacological properties, documented adverse effect profile, dose-response relationships, or patient risk factors. Examples include bleeding with anticoagulants, gastrointestinal effects with NSAIDs, or sedation with antihistamines. Such reactions are extensions of known pharmacology and generally dose-related.

Unpredictable (Type B) reactions: These cannot be anticipated from known pharmacology or existing product information. They typically represent immunological reactions, genetic idiosyncrasies, or novel mechanisms. Examples include anaphylaxis in previously unexposed individuals, drug-induced lupus, or idiosyncratic hepatotoxicity. These reactions are usually dose-independent and occur unpredictably.

Assessment of predictability helps in several ways: guiding patient education about potential effects to expect, informing monitoring strategies for high-risk patients, supporting causality assessment (predictable reactions have higher prior probability), and identifying novel reactions requiring scientific investigation and product information updates.

Preventability Assessment

Preventability evaluates whether the adverse reaction could have been avoided through different prescribing, dispensing, or administration practices. This assessment has major implications for quality improvement and patient safety initiatives.

Various tools exist for assessing preventability, but common criteria include:

Definite preventability: The reaction was clearly caused by errors or deviations from accepted practices, such as prescribing despite documented contraindications, ignoring serious drug-drug interactions, using inappropriate doses for patient's renal or hepatic function, failing to monitor when monitoring is clearly indicated, or continuing therapy despite early warning signs.

Probable preventability: The reaction likely could have been prevented through different practices, though judgment is involved. Examples include prescribing when safer alternatives existed, inadequate patient education about serious risks, marginal dose selection without adequate justification, or suboptimal monitoring.

Not preventable: The reaction occurred despite appropriate prescribing, monitoring, and patient care. This includes many unpredictable reactions, reactions in patients without identifiable risk factors, or reactions despite all reasonable precautions.

Applications in Healthcare Improvement

Preventability assessment serves multiple purposes. Individual case analysis identifies specific failures in medication management requiring corrective action. Aggregate analysis of preventability reveals systematic problems in prescribing practices, monitoring protocols, healthcare professional knowledge, medication system design, or patient education.

Quality improvement initiatives target preventable adverse reactions through interventions like clinical decision support systems, enhanced prescribing guidelines, improved patient education materials, medication reconciliation programs, and expanded therapeutic drug monitoring.

Educational programs for healthcare professionals emphasize prevention strategies, recognition of high-risk situations, appropriate monitoring protocols, and effective patient communication. Patients benefit from education about warning signs requiring immediate medical attention, proper medication administration, and importance of disclosing all medications and health conditions to prescribers.

2.11 MANAGEMENT OF ADVERSE DRUG REACTIONS

Effective management of adverse drug reactions requires prompt recognition, appropriate intervention, and measures to prevent recurrence. Management approaches vary based on reaction severity, mechanism, and clinical context.

Immediate Management

When an ADR is suspected, the first priority is assessing severity and need for urgent intervention. Life-threatening reactions require immediate emergency treatment - anaphylaxis demands epinephrine administration, airway management, and hemodynamic support; severe bleeding requires hemorrhage control and reversal agents; and serious arrhythmias need appropriate cardiac interventions.

Drug discontinuation is appropriate for serious reactions, when safer alternatives exist, or when risks clearly outweigh benefits. However, this decision requires careful judgment - abrupt discontinuation of some drugs (corticosteroids, beta-blockers, antiepileptics) carries its own risks necessitating gradual tapering.

Symptomatic treatment addresses reaction manifestations - antihistamines and corticosteroids for allergic reactions, antiemetics for nausea, analgesics for pain, or antidiarrheal agents for gastrointestinal disturbances.

Specific Interventions

Antidotes and reversal agents are available for certain drug toxicities: naloxone for opioid overdose, flumazenil for benzodiazepine toxicity, protamine for heparin reversal, vitamin K or specific factor concentrates for warfarin-associated bleeding, and chelating agents for heavy metal poisoning.

Dose reduction may suffice for dose-dependent reactions when drug therapy must continue. Careful dose adjustment based on patient characteristics, renal or hepatic function, and drug interactions can reduce adverse effect intensity while maintaining therapeutic benefit.

Supportive care including hydration, nutritional support, monitoring of vital signs and laboratory parameters, and prevention of complications forms the foundation of ADR management, particularly for reactions without specific treatments.

Long-Term Management

Alternative therapy should be identified when the offending drug must be discontinued. Selection considers cross-reactivity patterns (avoiding structurally similar compounds for immunological reactions), different mechanisms of action, and patient-specific factors affecting drug choice.

Patient education is crucial for preventing recurrence. Patients must understand which drugs to avoid, importance of disclosing ADR history to all healthcare providers, recognition of early warning signs, and wearing medical alert identification for serious allergies.

Documentation ensures information accessibility across healthcare settings. ADR history should be recorded prominently in medical records, electronic health records should include allergy alerts, and reporting to pharmacovigilance systems contributes to broader medication safety.

Follow-Up

Systematic follow-up ensures complete reaction resolution, identifies any persistent sequelae requiring ongoing management, provides opportunity for patient education reinforcement, and enables completion of ADR reports with outcome information. Long-term follow-up may be necessary for reactions with delayed manifestations or chronic consequences.

2.12 ECONOMIC BURDEN OF ADRs

Adverse drug reactions impose substantial economic costs on healthcare systems, patients, and society through direct medical expenses, indirect costs, and intangible impacts on quality of life.

Direct Medical Costs

Hospital admissions caused by ADRs represent a major cost driver. Studies across countries show that 3-10% of hospital admissions result from adverse drug reactions, with serious reactions more commonly necessitating hospitalization. The average cost per ADR-related hospitalization typically exceeds routine admissions due to medical complexity and longer stays.

Emergency department visits for managing acute adverse reactions add substantial costs, particularly for allergic reactions, overdoses, and drug interactions producing acute symptoms.

Prolonged hospital stays occur when ADRs develop during hospitalization, extending length of stay beyond that required for the primary condition. Each additional day incurs costs for accommodation, nursing care, and medical management.

Additional treatments required to manage adverse reactions include medications, procedures, laboratory testing, imaging studies, and sometimes surgical interventions. The cascade of interventions needed to address serious ADRs significantly multiplies costs.

Monitoring and prevention costs for high-risk medications include therapeutic drug monitoring, laboratory testing (renal function, liver enzymes, complete blood counts), and clinician time for assessment and management.

Indirect Economic Costs

Lost productivity from patients missing work, reduced work capacity during recovery, or permanent disability from serious ADRs represents substantial economic impact beyond direct medical costs. Caregivers may also require time off work to support affected patients.

Premature mortality from fatal adverse reactions causes loss of productive life years, with economic value extending beyond immediate medical costs to lifetime earning potential lost.

Litigation costs when ADRs result from medication errors or negligence include legal expenses, settlements, and damage awards, though these represent only a fraction of total ADR costs.

Healthcare System Impact

ADRs strain healthcare resources, diverting attention and resources from other patients and conditions. In resource-limited settings, the economic burden is particularly significant, potentially reducing capacity to provide other essential services.

Preventable ADRs represent avoidable costs to healthcare systems. Studies suggest 30-50% of adverse drug reactions are preventable through better prescribing, monitoring, and medication management practices. The economic burden of preventable ADRs highlights opportunities for cost-effective interventions.

Cost-Effectiveness of Prevention

Pharmacovigilance activities, despite requiring resources, are highly cost-effective by preventing adverse events through early signal detection, enabling targeted risk management, promoting rational prescribing, and informing clinical decision-making with safety data.

Interventions with demonstrated economic benefits include clinical pharmacist involvement in medication management, computerized prescriber order entry with decision support, medication reconciliation programs, and therapeutic drug monitoring for high-risk medications.

Table 5: Components of ADR Economic Burden

Cost Category	Components	Estimated Contribution
Direct Medical	Hospital admissions, ER visits, additional treatments, monitoring	50-60% of total costs
Indirect Economic	Lost productivity, disability, premature mortality	30-40% of total costs
Intangible	Pain, suffering, reduced quality of life	Not monetarily quantified
System Impact	Resource diversion, capacity reduction	Varies by healthcare system

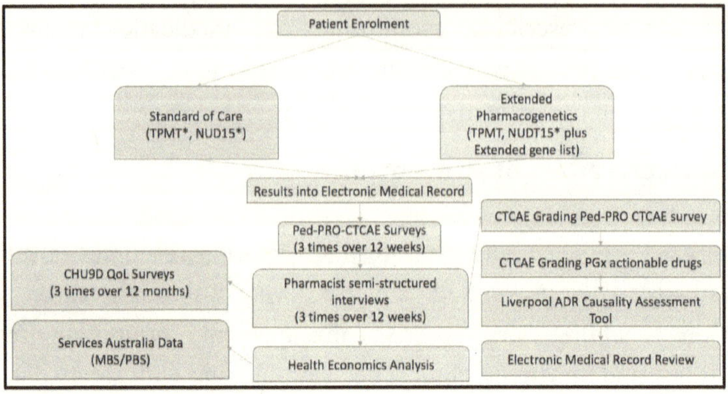

Figure 5: The economic burden of adverse drug reactions encompasses multiple cost categories extending beyond immediate medical expenses.

Global Perspective

Economic burden varies across countries based on healthcare system structure, drug utilization patterns, availability of pharmacovigilance infrastructure, and population demographics. However, the consistent finding globally is that ADRs impose substantial, largely preventable economic costs. Investment in pharmacovigilance, medication safety programs, and healthcare professional education offers high returns through reduced ADR incidence and associated costs.

The recognition of ADRs' economic impact has elevated medication safety as a healthcare priority, driving quality improvement initiatives, regulatory requirements for risk management plans, and allocation of resources to pharmacovigilance activities.

Adverse drug reactions represent a significant clinical, public health, and economic challenge requiring systematic understanding, detection, assessment, and management. Precise terminology and classification systems including Rawlins and Thompson's Type A/Type B framework and the more comprehensive DoTS system facilitate communication and guide clinical approaches. Standardized causality assessment tools like the WHO-UMC scale and Naranjo Algorithm improve consistency in determining drug-event relationships, while severity, seriousness, predictability, and preventability assessments inform clinical decisions and regulatory priorities.

Effective ADR management requires prompt recognition, appropriate intervention ranging from symptomatic treatment to specific antidotes, and preventive measures to avoid recurrence. The substantial economic burden imposed by adverse reactions - through direct medical costs, indirect productivity losses, and healthcare system impacts - underscores the value of robust pharmacovigilance systems. Understanding that many ADRs are preventable through optimal prescribing, monitoring, and medication management emphasizes the importance of healthcare professional education, clinical decision support, and continuous safety monitoring throughout the medication lifecycle.

The foundation established in this chapter - encompassing definitions, classifications, detection methods, assessment tools, and management principles - provides the essential framework for advanced pharmacovigilance practice explored in subsequent chapters.

CHAPTER 3

BASIC TERMINOLOGIES USED IN PHARMACOVIGILANCE

KEY OUTCOMES

Upon completion of this chapter, learners will be able to:

1. Define and differentiate various adverse medication-related event terminologies
2. Explain the concept of suspected adverse reactions and reporting criteria
3. Distinguish between expected and unexpected adverse reactions
4. Understand the concept and significance of signals in pharmacovigilance
5. Differentiate between medical errors and medication errors with examples
6. Explain regulatory terminologies: IND, NDA, and ANDA
7. Describe the roles and responsibilities of Marketing Authorization Holders
8. Apply risk-benefit analysis principles in medication safety assessment
9. Understand off-label drug use and its pharmacovigilance implications

ABSTRACT

Standardized terminology forms the essential foundation for effective pharmacovigilance communication, data collection, analysis, and regulatory compliance across international boundaries. This chapter provides comprehensive coverage of fundamental terminologies used in pharmacovigilance practice, encompassing adverse medication-related events, signal detection concepts, medication errors, and regulatory terms critical for drug development and post-marketing surveillance. Beginning with precise definitions of suspected and unexpected adverse reactions, the chapter explores the concept of signals in pharmacovigilance and distinguishes between medical errors and medication errors. Regulatory terminologies including IND, NDA, and ANDA are explained within their procedural contexts, while concepts such as Marketing Authorization Holder responsibilities, risk-benefit analysis frameworks, and off-label drug use are examined for their pharmacovigilance implications. Mastery of these standardized terms enables clear communication among healthcare professionals, regulatory authorities, pharmaceutical industry, and international pharmacovigilance networks.

3.1 TERMINOLOGIES OF ADVERSE MEDICATION-RELATED EVENTS

Pharmacovigilance employs specific terminology to categorize and communicate various types of adverse medication-related events. Precise use of these terms ensures clarity in reporting, analysis, and regulatory decision-making.

Adverse Event (AE)

An adverse event is any untoward medical occurrence in a patient administered a pharmaceutical product, which does not necessarily have a causal relationship with the treatment. The key characteristic is temporal association rather than proven causality. Any medical problem occurring during drug therapy qualifies as an adverse event regardless of whether the drug caused it.

This broad definition is particularly important in clinical trials where all adverse events must be documented, allowing subsequent analysis to determine which events represent true adverse drug reactions. In post-marketing surveillance, the term encompasses all reported occurrences, acknowledging that causality assessment occurs after initial reporting.

Adverse Drug Reaction (ADR)

An adverse drug reaction represents a subset of adverse events where a causal relationship between the drug and the event is suspected or established. The WHO definition specifies that ADRs are noxious and unintended responses occurring at doses normally used for prophylaxis, diagnosis, therapy, or physiological function modification.

The distinction between adverse events and adverse drug reactions is crucial: all ADRs are adverse events, but not all adverse events are ADRs. For example, if a patient taking an antibiotic develops pneumonia, this is an adverse event but likely not an ADR unless an immunological or other drug-related mechanism is suspected.

Adverse Reaction

Adverse reaction is often used interchangeably with adverse drug reaction, referring to harmful or unintended responses to medicines. In regulatory contexts, the term emphasizes that some level of causal relationship is suspected or established, distinguishing it from the broader adverse event category.

Side Effect

A side effect represents any unintended effect of a pharmaceutical product occurring at normal doses, which may be beneficial, neutral, or harmful. Not all side effects are adverse - some may be therapeutically exploited. For instance, the sedative side effect of antihistamines, while adverse when driving is required, becomes therapeutically useful when treating insomnia.

The term "side effect" is commonly used in patient communication and product labeling to describe known, generally minor or expected effects that accompany therapeutic action. In technical pharmacovigilance terminology, the more specific term "adverse drug reaction" is preferred when effects are harmful.

Serious Adverse Event (SAE)

A serious adverse event meets specific regulatory criteria regardless of causality assessment. An event qualifies as serious if it results in death, is life-threatening, requires hospitalization or prolongation of existing hospitalization, results in persistent or significant disability/incapacity, is a congenital anomaly/birth defect, or is a medically important event requiring intervention to prevent serious outcomes.

The regulatory definition of seriousness drives reporting timelines and regulatory obligations. Serious adverse events from clinical trials must be reported to regulatory authorities within specified timeframes (typically 7-15 days for fatal or life-threatening events).

Unexpected Adverse Reaction

An unexpected adverse reaction is one whose nature, severity, or outcome is not consistent with the reference safety information. For marketed products, reference information is the approved product label. In clinical trials, it refers to the investigator's brochure or protocol safety information.

Unexpectedness is determined not by whether the reaction could theoretically occur, but whether it is documented in current product information. A known reaction occurring with greater frequency or severity than previously documented may also qualify as unexpected.

3.2 SUSPECTED ADVERSE REACTION

A suspected adverse reaction is an adverse event for which there is a reasonable possibility of a causal relationship between the drug and the event, based on available information. The concept of "suspected" acknowledges uncertainty inherent in pharmacovigilance - definitive proof of causality is often impossible, yet precautionary reporting serves public health interests.

Criteria for Suspicion

Several factors support suspicion of causality: appropriate temporal relationship between drug administration and event onset; known pharmacological properties consistent with the reaction; absence of more likely alternative explanations; positive dechallenge (improvement after drug discontinuation); or previous reports of similar reactions with the drug or related compounds.

Healthcare professionals need not establish definitive causality before reporting - suspicion based on clinical judgment suffices. The principle "when in doubt, report" underlies effective pharmacovigilance, as expert assessment occurs centrally after report collection.

Reporting Obligations

Healthcare professionals should report suspected adverse reactions, particularly those that are serious, unexpected, or occurring with new medicines. Pharmaceutical companies have legal obligations to report all suspected adverse reactions that come to their attention through any source including spontaneous reports, clinical trials, literature, and post-marketing studies.

Clinical Context

In clinical practice, suspected adverse reactions require clinical judgment balancing patient safety with therapeutic benefit. Management decisions depend on reaction severity, availability of alternatives, and patient-specific factors. Documentation ensures the suspected reaction is considered in future prescribing decisions for that patient and contributes to pharmacovigilance databases.

3.3 UNEXPECTED ADVERSE REACTION

Unexpected adverse reactions are those not previously observed or documented in current reference safety information, or that occur with greater severity, frequency, or different characteristics than previously described.

Determination of Expectedness

For marketed medicines, the approved product labeling (package insert, summary of product characteristics) serves as reference information. Any reaction not listed in these documents is considered unexpected. For investigational drugs in clinical trials, the investigator's brochure or protocol safety information defines expected reactions.

Unexpectedness encompasses several scenarios: completely novel reactions never before associated with the drug; known reactions occurring with greater frequency than documented; known reactions with greater severity than previously described; or known reactions with altered characteristics (different patient populations, different outcomes).

Regulatory Significance

Unexpected adverse reactions trigger expedited reporting requirements. Serious, unexpected suspected adverse reactions (SUSARs) from clinical trials must be reported to regulatory authorities within 7-15 days, depending on whether the event was fatal or life-threatening. This expedited reporting enables rapid regulatory assessment and protective action if needed.

For marketed products, unexpected serious adverse reactions may prompt regulatory review of product labeling, risk management plans, or even market withdrawal depending on severity and frequency. The distinction between expected and unexpected reactions drives regulatory scrutiny and communication priorities.

Evolution of Expectedness

As drugs are used more extensively and knowledge accumulates, reactions initially considered unexpected become expected through documentation in updated product information. This dynamic process reflects pharmacovigilance's continuous learning model - new information constantly refines understanding of drug safety profiles.

3.4 SIGNAL IN PHARMACOVIGILANCE

A signal represents information arising from one or multiple sources suggesting a new potential causal association, or a new aspect of a known association, between an intervention and an event or set of related events that is judged to be of sufficient likelihood to justify verificatory action.

Signal Characteristics

Signals represent hypotheses requiring verification rather than established facts. They emerge from various sources including spontaneous reporting systems, clinical trial data, epidemiological studies, literature reports, or laboratory findings. The key characteristic is that the information suggests a previously unrecognized hazard or new understanding of a known hazard.

Quantitative signals arise from statistical analysis of large databases, identifying disproportionate reporting patterns. If a particular drug-event combination is reported more frequently than expected based on overall reporting patterns, this disproportionality constitutes a signal requiring evaluation.

Qualitative signals emerge from individual case reports or small series demonstrating distinctive features suggesting causality, such as positive rechallenge, characteristic dose-response relationships, or specific laboratory findings.

Signal Detection Methods

Spontaneous reporting analysis employs statistical algorithms to identify disproportionate reporting. Methods include Proportional Reporting Ratio (PRR), Reporting Odds Ratio (ROR), and Bayesian approaches like Empirical Bayes Geometric Mean (EBGM). These methods compare observed versus expected reporting frequencies.

Data mining techniques systematically screen large safety databases for unusual patterns or associations. Automated algorithms can process millions of reports to identify potential signals requiring expert review.

Clinical review of individual case reports, particularly those demonstrating strong causality evidence, distinctive clinical features, or occurring in unexpected populations, generates signals through qualitative assessment.

Literature surveillance involves systematic monitoring of scientific and medical publications for case reports, case series, or study results suggesting new safety concerns.

Signal Evaluation

Once detected, signals undergo rigorous evaluation to determine whether they represent true drug safety issues. Evaluation considers biological plausibility, strength of evidence from case reports, epidemiological data when available, consistency across different data sources, and impact assessment regarding frequency and severity.

Signal validation determines whether sufficient evidence exists to conclude a causal association is likely. Signal prioritization ranks validated signals by public health importance, considering severity, frequency, preventability, and affected populations.

Signal Management

Validated signals trigger actions proportionate to the risk identified. Actions may include regulatory communications to healthcare professionals, product labeling updates, implementation of risk minimization measures, requirements for additional studies, or in severe cases, market restriction or withdrawal.

Table 6: Signal Detection and Management Process

Stage	Activities	Outcome
Signal Detection	Statistical analysis, clinical review, literature surveillance	Potential signal identified
Signal Validation	Causality assessment, evidence evaluation, biological plausibility review	Confirmed or refuted signal
Signal Prioritization	Public health impact assessment, frequency and severity analysis	Priority ranking for action
Signal Management	Regulatory communication, labeling updates, risk minimization, further studies	Implemented protective measures

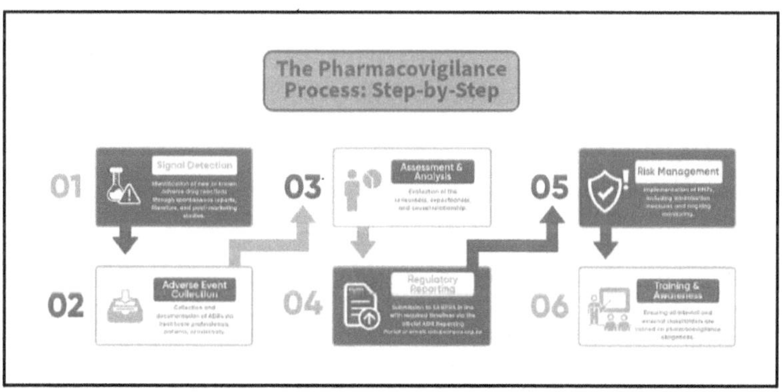

Figure. 6: The signal management process in pharmacovigilance follows a systematic pathway from initial detection through validation, prioritization, and ultimately to implementation of appropriate protective measures.

3.5 MEDICAL ERROR AND MEDICATION ERROR

Understanding the distinction between medical errors and medication errors is essential for comprehensive patient safety monitoring and appropriate preventive interventions.

Medical Error

A medical error is a preventable adverse event that occurs as a result of healthcare management rather than an underlying disease. Medical errors encompass mistakes in any aspect of healthcare delivery including diagnosis, treatment, disease management, preventive care, and health system operations.

Medical errors may involve incorrect diagnoses, surgical errors, wrong-site surgery, healthcare-associated infections, communication failures, delays in treatment, or equipment failures. These errors span all healthcare disciplines and settings.

Medication Error

A medication error is a specific type of medical error involving medicines, defined as any preventable event that may cause or lead to inappropriate medication use or patient harm while the medication is in control of healthcare professional, patient, or consumer. These errors occur at any stage of the medication use process.

Types of Medication Errors

Prescribing errors involve incorrect drug selection, inappropriate dosing, failure to consider contraindications, drug interactions, or patient-specific factors like renal or hepatic function. Examples include prescribing penicillin to patients with documented allergy, inappropriate doses for elderly patients, or drugs contraindicated with concurrent conditions.

Dispensing errors occur in pharmacies when incorrect medicines are provided, wrong doses dispensed, incorrect labels applied, or inadequate patient counseling provided. These errors may involve look-alike/sound-alike drug confusion or misreading of prescriptions.

Administration errors happen when drugs are given via wrong routes, at incorrect times, in wrong doses, to wrong patients, or with inappropriate administration techniques. Common in hospitals, these errors often result from communication breakdowns or workflow interruptions.

Monitoring errors involve failure to review therapy appropriately, inadequate therapeutic drug monitoring, missed laboratory checks, or failure to recognize and respond to adverse effects. These errors allow preventable harm to continue unrecognized.

Patient adherence errors include taking incorrect doses, wrong timing, premature discontinuation, or inappropriate medication sharing. While sometimes classified separately from healthcare system errors, they represent important safety concerns requiring intervention through education and support.

Consequences of Medication Errors

Medication errors may result in actual adverse drug events causing patient harm, or may be intercepted before reaching the patient (potential adverse drug events). Even errors not causing harm provide valuable learning opportunities for system improvement.

The Institute of Medicine's landmark report "To Err is Human" highlighted that medication errors contribute significantly to healthcare-related injuries and deaths, with many being preventable through system improvements.

Prevention Strategies

System-level interventions include computerized physician order entry (CPOE) with clinical decision support, barcode medication administration systems, standardized protocols and checklists, improved medication packaging and labeling, and separation of look-alike/sound-alike medications.

Professional-level interventions involve continuing education on high-risk medications and populations, double-check procedures for high-alert drugs, effective communication protocols, and adequate staffing to prevent workload-related errors.

Patient-level interventions encompass medication reconciliation at transitions of care, patient education about proper medication use, encouraging patients to question and report concerns, and simplified medication regimens when possible.

3.6 REGULATORY TERMINOLOGIES

Understanding regulatory terminology is essential for navigating drug development, approval processes, and post-marketing obligations within pharmacovigilance frameworks.

Regulatory Authority

A regulatory authority (also called medicines agency or drug regulatory agency) is the government body responsible for regulating pharmaceuticals within a specific jurisdiction. Examples include the US Food and Drug Administration (FDA), European Medicines Agency (EMA), Medicines and Healthcare products Regulatory Agency (MHRA) in UK, and Central Drugs Standard Control Organization (CDSCO) in India.

Regulatory authorities evaluate new drug applications, approve medicines for marketing, monitor post-marketing safety, enforce regulations, and take action when safety concerns arise including label changes or market withdrawals.

Marketing Authorization

Marketing authorization (also called marketing approval, product license, or drug registration) is official permission granted by regulatory authorities allowing a pharmaceutical company to market a medicine in a specific territory. Authorization is granted after reviewing evidence of quality, safety, and efficacy.Marketing authorization typically specifies approved indications, dosage forms, strengths, patient populations, and conditions of use. Post-marketing obligations often accompany authorization, including periodic safety reports and commitments to conduct additional studies.

Pharmacopoeia

A pharmacopoeia is an official compendium containing standards for medicines including specifications for identity, purity, strength, and quality. Major pharmacopoeias include the United States Pharmacopeia (USP), British Pharmacopoeia (BP), European Pharmacopoeia (EP), and Indian Pharmacopoeia (IP).

Compliance with pharmacopoeial standards is typically required for marketing authorization. These standards ensure product quality and consistency, supporting patient safety and therapeutic effectiveness.

Good Pharmacovigilance Practices (GVP)

Good Pharmacovigilance Practices represent standards and guidelines for performing pharmacovigilance activities. The European Medicines Agency has published comprehensive GVP modules covering all aspects from quality systems through risk management. These practices ensure systematic, consistent, high-quality pharmacovigilance.

Competent Authority

A competent authority is the regulatory body responsible for specific regulatory functions within a jurisdiction. In pharmacovigilance, the competent authority receives safety reports, evaluates signals, and implements regulatory actions. The term is commonly used in European contexts where individual member states have their own competent authorities coordinating with the EMA.

3.7 IND, NDA, ANDA DEFINITIONS

These acronyms represent critical stages and pathways in drug development and approval processes in the United States, with analogous procedures in other regulatory systems.

Investigational New Drug Application (IND)

An IND is a request for authorization from the FDA to administer an investigational drug to humans in clinical trials. Before any clinical testing in humans can begin, sponsors must submit an IND containing preclinical data demonstrating reasonable safety, manufacturing information ensuring quality, and proposed clinical trial protocols.

The IND process enables FDA oversight of clinical investigations, ensuring patient protection through review of study protocols, informed consent documents, and ongoing safety monitoring. Sponsors must submit annual reports and safety updates throughout the investigational period.

Three types exist: Commercial IND submitted by companies intending to market the drug; Research IND submitted by academic or research investigators; and Treatment IND allowing use of investigational drugs for seriously ill patients outside clinical trials under specific circumstances.

New Drug Application (NDA)

An NDA is the formal request to the FDA for approval to market a new drug for human use in the United States. The NDA represents the culmination of drug development, submitted after completing preclinical studies and adequate, well-controlled clinical trials demonstrating safety and efficacy.

The NDA must contain comprehensive data including chemistry and manufacturing information, nonclinical pharmacology and toxicology studies, human pharmacokinetics and bioavailability studies, clinical efficacy and safety data, proposed labeling, and a risk-benefit analysis. The FDA review process typically takes 10-12 months for standard applications.

Approval grants the sponsor marketing authorization for specified indications, with requirements for post-marketing surveillance, periodic safety update reports, and sometimes post-marketing studies addressing remaining questions about safety or efficacy.

Abbreviated New Drug Application (ANDA)

An ANDA is the application for approval of generic drugs in the United States. Unlike NDAs requiring full preclinical and clinical data, ANDAs allow approval based primarily on demonstrating pharmaceutical equivalence and bioequivalence to an approved reference listed drug (the original brand-name product).

ANDAs must show the generic drug contains the same active ingredient(s) in the same strength and dosage form, is bioequivalent to the reference product, meets quality standards, and is manufactured according to good manufacturing practices. Clinical efficacy studies are not required - bioequivalence serves as the bridge to the reference product's established safety and efficacy.

Generic drug approval expands treatment access and reduces costs while maintaining standards through bioequivalence requirements. Post-marketing pharmacovigilance for generic drugs follows similar principles to innovator products, with manufacturers required to report adverse events and comply with regulatory requirements.

3.8 MARKETING AUTHORIZATION HOLDER (MAH)

The Marketing Authorization Holder (also called market authorization holder, product license holder, or in some regions, the applicant or sponsor) is the person or legal entity that has been granted marketing authorization for a medicinal product by the regulatory authority.

Responsibilities

The MAH holds ultimate responsibility for the medicine throughout its lifecycle. Quality responsibilities include ensuring manufacturing complies with good manufacturing practices, maintaining product quality specifications, managing supply chain integrity, and implementing quality systems for deviation management and corrective actions.

Pharmacovigilance obligations are extensive. The MAH must establish and maintain a pharmacovigilance system, appoint a qualified person responsible for pharmacovigilance, collect and report adverse events according to regulatory timelines, submit periodic safety update reports, conduct signal detection and risk assessment, and implement risk minimization measures when needed.

Regulatory compliance requires maintaining current product information, submitting variation applications for changes, complying with post-authorization commitments, responding to regulatory requests, and ensuring promotional materials are accurate and balanced.

Pharmacovigilance System

The MAH must establish a robust pharmacovigilance system encompassing organizational structures with clear responsibilities, standard operating procedures for all pharmacovigilance activities, quality systems ensuring data integrity and compliance, information technology systems for case processing and reporting, and adequate resources including trained personnel.

A Qualified Person Responsible for Pharmacovigilance (QPPV) must be appointed by the MAH. The QPPV oversees the pharmacovigilance system, ensures compliance with regulatory requirements, serves as the contact point with authorities, and maintains oversight of all pharmacovigilance activities globally.

Risk Management

MAHs must develop and implement Risk Management Plans (RMPs) for new medicines and sometimes for established products with emerging safety concerns. RMPs include safety specifications describing known and potential risks, pharmacovigilance plans for monitoring risks, and risk minimization measures to prevent or reduce risk occurrence or severity.

Table 7: MAH Pharmacovigilance Responsibilities

Responsibility Area	Key Activities	Regulatory Impact
System Establishment	Appoint QPPV, establish SOPs, maintain databases	Foundation for all PV activities
Case Management	Collect, process, assess, and report adverse events	Compliance with reporting timelines
Signal Detection	Monitor safety data, identify and evaluate signals	Early identification of safety concerns
Risk Management	Develop RMPs, implement risk minimization measures	Proactive safety management
Regulatory Reporting	Submit PSURs/PBRERs, respond to authority requests	Ongoing authorization maintenance

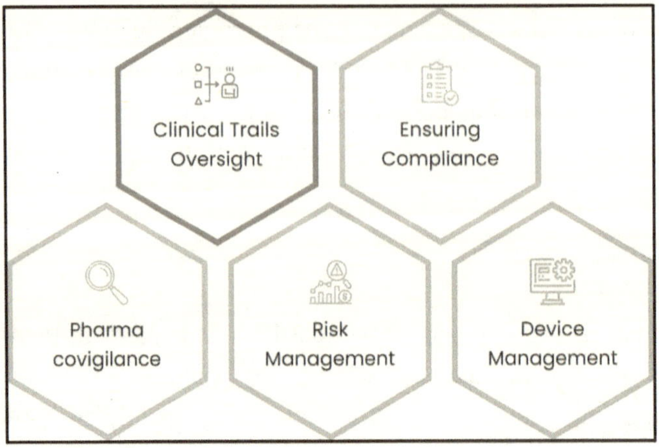
Clinical Trails Oversight
Ensuring Compliance
Pharma covigilance
Risk Management
Device Management

Figure 7: Marketing Authorization Holders bear comprehensive responsibilities spanning the entire lifecycle of their products.

3.9 RISK-BENEFIT ANALYSIS

Risk-benefit analysis is the systematic evaluation of favorable effects (benefits) against unfavorable effects (risks) of a medical intervention, forming the foundation for regulatory decisions and clinical practice.

Concept and Importance

No medicine is completely without risk. The fundamental principle underlying medicine regulation and use is that benefits must outweigh risks for approved indications in target populations when used according to recommendations. This balance is dynamic rather than static - new information may shift the balance over time.

Risk-benefit analysis guides multiple decisions: regulatory authorities determine whether to approve new medicines, approve label changes, or withdraw marketing authorization; prescribers decide whether to prescribe for individual patients; and patients make informed decisions about accepting treatment.

Components of Risk Assessment

Identification of risks includes all potential adverse effects from mild to severe, considering frequency, severity, reversibility, and preventability. Both common mild reactions and rare serious reactions contribute to overall risk profile.

Characterization of risks evaluates the nature of adverse effects, populations at higher risk, dose-relationships, temporal patterns, and impact on quality of life. Risk characterization provides detailed understanding beyond simple identification.

Quantification of risks involves determining frequency of adverse effects, typically expressed as incidence rates (number of new cases per person-time) or prevalence. Rare events (1 in 10,000) carry different weight than common events (1 in 10), though severity also matters.

Components of Benefit Assessment

Efficacy data from clinical trials demonstrate whether the medicine produces intended therapeutic effects under controlled conditions. Endpoints may be clinical outcomes (mortality, symptom resolution), surrogate markers (blood pressure reduction, cholesterol lowering), or quality of life improvements.

Effectiveness data from real-world use shows whether therapeutic benefits observed in trials translate to routine clinical practice across diverse patient populations and settings.

Magnitude of benefit considers size of treatment effect, proportion of patients experiencing benefit, time to benefit onset, and duration of benefit. Modest benefits may suffice for serious conditions lacking alternatives, while substantial benefits are expected for less serious conditions with existing treatments.

Balance Evaluation

The risk-benefit balance is indication-specific - acceptable risks for life-threatening cancer may be unacceptable for mild headaches.

Population-specific factors influence balance - age, disease severity, comorbidities, pregnancy status, and concurrent medications affect both risks and benefits.

Alternative therapies availability influences acceptable risk - higher risks may be tolerable when no alternatives exist, while effective, safer alternatives narrow the acceptable risk profile.

Patient perspectives on risk tolerance, quality of life priorities, and treatment goals inform individualized risk-benefit decisions in clinical practice, though regulatory decisions consider population-level benefits and risks.

Evolution Over Time

Risk-benefit balance evolves as new information emerges. Post-marketing surveillance may identify previously unknown risks, reveal benefits in new populations, or show different real-world effectiveness than clinical trials suggested. Periodic reassessment ensures the balance remains favorable, prompting label updates, usage restrictions, or market withdrawals when necessary.

3.10 OFF-LABEL USE

Off-label use refers to the use of a medicine for an indication, in a dosage, or for a population not included in the approved product labeling. This practice is common, legal in most jurisdictions for prescribers, yet carries specific implications for pharmacovigilance and regulatory oversight.

Definition and Scope

Off-label use encompasses several scenarios: prescribing for unapproved indications (e.g., using antidepressants for neuropathic pain), using different doses than approved (e.g., higher-than-approved doses), treating populations not included in approval (e.g., pediatric use when only approved for adults), or using different routes of administration.

The extent of off-label prescribing varies by therapeutic area and specialty. In oncology and pediatrics, off-label use is particularly common due to limited approved options and the impracticality of conducting trials for every possible use in every population.

Legal and Ethical Considerations

In most countries, prescribers legally may prescribe approved medicines for off-label uses based on their medical judgment and available evidence. This flexibility enables innovation and addresses patient needs when approved alternatives are inadequate. However, prescribers bear responsibility for ensuring their off-label use is evidence-based and in patients' best interests.

Pharmaceutical companies face strict restrictions - they generally cannot promote medicines for off-label uses, as such promotion could circumvent regulatory approval processes designed to ensure evidence of safety and efficacy. Violations can result in substantial penalties.

Informed consent takes on particular importance for off-label use. Patients should understand when medicines are prescribed outside approved indications, the evidence supporting such use, and that safety data may be more limited than for approved uses.

Evidence Base

Off-label uses exist on a spectrum of evidence. Some off-label uses have robust evidence from well-designed studies and are supported by clinical practice guidelines, representing standard-of-care despite lacking formal approval. Others rely on limited case reports, small studies, or theoretical rationale, representing more experimental uses.

The lack of approval does not necessarily mean lack of efficacy - often medicines are not approved for all effective uses simply because manufacturers have not pursued approval (due to expired patents, small markets, or other commercial considerations).

Pharmacovigilance Implications

Off-label use creates specific challenges and considerations for pharmacovigilance. Safety data limitations arise because pre-marketing studies focused on approved indications may not represent off-label uses. Different indications may involve different patient populations, doses, or durations of therapy, potentially revealing distinct safety profiles.

Reporting considerations require that adverse events from off-label use be reported to pharmacovigilance systems just as for approved uses. However, causality assessment may be complicated when use differs substantially from approved parameters.

Regulatory monitoring of widespread off-label use may prompt regulatory authorities to request additional safety data or encourage manufacturers to pursue formal approval for common off-label indications, ensuring systematic evaluation and appropriate labeling.

Pediatric Off-Label Use

Children represent a special case where off-label use is particularly prevalent due to limited pediatric trials and approvals. Many medicines are used in children based on extrapolation from adult data, with dosing adjusted by weight or body surface area. This practice, while often necessary, creates uncertainty about safety and efficacy in developing bodies with different pharmacokinetics and pharmacodynamics.

Regulatory initiatives in various countries provide incentives for pediatric studies, gradually reducing but not eliminating pediatric off-label use. Enhanced pharmacovigilance for pediatric medicine use remains crucial given their vulnerability and limited evidence base.

Risk Management

Appropriate risk management for off-label use involves several elements: ensuring prescribers are informed about evidence quality and limitations, enhanced monitoring for adverse effects in off-label uses, clear patient communication about off-label status, documentation of rationale and informed consent, and systematic collection of safety and efficacy data to build evidence.

Healthcare institutions may implement formulary controls or protocols governing high-risk off-label uses, balancing innovation and patient access with safety concerns.

Mastery of pharmacovigilance terminology provides the essential foundation for effective communication, accurate reporting, and appropriate regulatory compliance across the diverse stakeholders involved in medication safety monitoring. The precise definitions distinguishing adverse events from adverse drug reactions, unexpected from expected reactions, and medical errors from medication errors enable clear documentation and systematic analysis of safety data. Understanding signals—their detection, validation, and management - forms the core of proactive pharmacovigilance identifying previously unrecognized hazards.

Regulatory terminologies including IND, NDA, and ANDA situate pharmacovigilance within the broader drug development and approval framework, while the concept of Marketing Authorization Holder delineates accountability for ongoing safety monitoring. Risk-benefit analysis provides the conceptual foundation for all regulatory and clinical decisions regarding medicine use, recognizing that perfect safety is unattainable and benefits must be balanced against inevitable risks. Finally, off-label use highlights the complexity of real-world medicine use extending beyond approved indications, with specific implications for pharmacovigilance monitoring and evidence generation.

These standardized terminologies, recognized internationally and applied consistently across regulatory authorities, pharmaceutical industry, healthcare providers, and research communities, enable the global collaboration essential for protecting public health in an increasingly interconnected world where medicines cross borders and safety information must be shared rapidly and unambiguously.

CHAPTER 4

DRUG AND DISEASE CLASSIFICATION

KEY OUTCOMES

Upon completion of this chapter, learners will be able to:

1. Understand the principles and structure of the Anatomical Therapeutic Chemical (ATC) classification system
2. Describe the five-level hierarchical structure of ATC codes and their application in pharmacovigilance
3. Explain the International Classification of Diseases (ICD) and its evolution from ICD-10 to ICD-11
4. Define Defined Daily Dose (DDD) and its significance in drug utilization studies
5. Understand the International Non-proprietary Names (INN) system and the WHO INN Programme
6. Apply classification systems for accurate coding in adverse drug reaction reporting
7. Recognize the importance of standardized nomenclature in global pharmacovigilance

ABSTRACT

This chapter provides a comprehensive understanding of international drug and disease classification systems that form the backbone of pharmacovigilance data management and regulatory reporting. The Anatomical Therapeutic Chemical (ATC) classification system offers a standardized method for categorizing pharmaceutical substances based on their therapeutic, pharmacological, and chemical properties. The International Classification of Diseases (ICD) provides a universal framework for coding and classifying diseases, injuries, and health conditions. Understanding these classification systems, along with concepts such as Defined Daily Dose (DDD) and International Non-proprietary Names (INN), is essential for accurate drug safety monitoring, adverse event reporting, and international regulatory harmonization. This chapter systematically explains the structure, application, and significance of these classification tools in pharmacovigilance practice.

4.1 ANATOMICAL THERAPEUTIC CHEMICAL (ATC) CLASSIFICATION OF DRUGS

The Anatomical Therapeutic Chemical (ATC) classification system is a globally recognized method for classifying pharmaceutical substances maintained by the World Health Organization Collaborating Centre for Drug Statistics Methodology (WHOCC). This system provides a standardized framework for categorizing drugs based on the organ or system they act upon and their therapeutic, pharmacological, and chemical properties.

The primary purpose of the ATC classification is to facilitate drug utilization studies, pharmacoepidemiological research, and pharmacovigilance activities. By providing a universal language for drug classification, the ATC system enables meaningful comparisons of drug consumption patterns across different countries, healthcare settings, and time periods. In pharmacovigilance, the ATC classification helps organize adverse drug reaction data, identify drug classes with similar safety profiles, and conduct signal detection activities.

The ATC system was first published by the European Pharmaceutical Market Research Association (EPhMRA) in 1976 and was subsequently adopted by the WHO. Since then, it has become the international standard for drug classification in drug utilization research and is widely used in pharmacovigilance databases, regulatory submissions, and scientific publications. The system is continuously updated to include new therapeutic substances and reflect advances in pharmacotherapy.

The fundamental principle of the ATC classification is that each drug substance is assigned a unique code based on its main therapeutic use. When a drug has multiple therapeutic applications, it receives several ATC codes corresponding to its different indications. For example, acetylsalicylic acid (aspirin) has different ATC codes when used as an analgesic-antipyretic (N02BA01), an antiplatelet agent (B01AC06), or an antirheumatic (M01BA03).

The ATC classification divides drug substances into different groups according to the organ or system on which they act and their therapeutic, pharmacological, and chemical properties. This hierarchical structure allows for classification at different levels of specificity, from broad anatomical groups to specific chemical substances.

4.2 STRUCTURE OF ATC CODES

The ATC classification system employs a five-level hierarchical structure, with each level providing progressively more specific information about the drug substance. This hierarchical organization facilitates both broad categorization and precise identification of pharmaceutical substances.

First Level: Anatomical Main Group (1 letter)

The first level consists of 14 main anatomical or pharmacological groups, each designated by a single letter. These main groups represent the organ system or body function upon which the drug acts.

The 14 main anatomical groups are:

- A – Alimentary tract and metabolism
- B – Blood and blood-forming organs
- C – Cardiovascular system
- D – Dermatologicals
- G – Genitourinary system and sex hormones
- H – Systemic hormonal preparations (excluding sex hormones and insulins)
- J – Antiinfectives for systemic use
- L – Antineoplastic and immunomodulating agents
- M – Musculoskeletal system
- N – Nervous system
- P – Antiparasitic products, insecticides, and repellents
- R – Respiratory system
- S – Sensory organs
- V – Various

Second Level: Therapeutic Subgroup (2 digits)

The second level provides a therapeutic or pharmacological subgroup within each main anatomical group. This level narrows down the classification to specific therapeutic categories.

For example, within group C (Cardiovascular system):

- C01 – Cardiac therapy
- C02 – Antihypertensives
- C03 – Diuretics
- C07 – Beta-blocking agents
- C09 – Agents acting on the renin-angiotensin system

Third Level: Pharmacological Subgroup (1 letter)

The third level specifies the pharmacological or therapeutic subgroup, providing further detail about the mechanism of action or therapeutic application.

For example, within C09 (Agents acting on the renin-angiotensin system):

- C09A – ACE inhibitors, plain
- C09B – ACE inhibitors, combinations
- C09C – Angiotensin II receptor blockers, plain
- C09D – Angiotensin II receptor blockers, combinations

Fourth Level: Chemical Subgroup (1 letter)

The fourth level identifies the chemical, therapeutic, or pharmacological subgroup, providing information about the chemical structure or specific therapeutic action.

For example, within C09C (Angiotensin II receptor blockers, plain):

- C09CA – Angiotensin II receptor blockers, plain

Fifth Level: Chemical Substance (2 digits)

The fifth and final level identifies the specific chemical substance. Each individual drug substance receives a unique two-digit code at this level.

For example, within C09CA:

- C09CA01 – Losartan
- C09CA02 – Eprosartan
- C09CA03 – Valsartan
- C09CA04 – Irbesartan
- C09CA06 – Candesartan
- C09CA07 – Telmisartan
- C09CA08 – Olmesartan medoxomil

Complete ATC Code Example

Let us examine the complete ATC code for Atorvastatin:

C10AA05

- C – Cardiovascular system (1st level)
- C10 – Lipid-modifying agents (2nd level)
- C10A – Lipid-modifying agents, plain (3rd level)
- C10AA – HMG CoA reductase inhibitors (4th level)
- C10AA05 – Atorvastatin (5th level)

This hierarchical structure allows pharmacovigilance professionals to analyze adverse drug reactions at various levels of specificity - from individual substances to entire therapeutic classes.

Table 8: Examples of Complete ATC Codes

Drug Substance	**ATC Code**	**Level 1**	**Level 2**	**Level 3**	**Level 4**	**Level 5**
Metformin	A10BA02	A (Alimentary)	A10 (Antidiabetics)	A10B (Blood glucose lowering drugs)	A10BA (Biguanides)	A10BA02 (Metformin)
Amoxicillin	J01CA04	J (Antiinfectives)	J01 (Antibacterials)	J01C (Beta-lactam antibacterials, penicillins)	J01CA (Penicillins with extended spectrum)	J01CA04 (Amoxicillin)
Omeprazole	A02BC01	A (Alimentary)	A02 (Drugs for acid-related disorders)	A02B (Drugs for peptic ulcer)	A02BC (Proton pump inhibitors)	A02BC01 (Omeprazole)

Level 2	Level 3	Level 4	Level 5	Example
C08 - Calcium channel blockers	C08C - Selective calcium channel blockers	C08CA - Selective calcium channel blockers with mainly vascular effects	C08CA01	Amlodipine
A10 - Drugs used in diabetes	A10B - Drugs used in diabetes excl. insulin	A10B - Drugs used in diabetes, excl. insulin	A10BA02	Metformin
N06 - Psycho-analeptic	N06A - Antide-presants	N06AB - Selective serotonin reuptake inhibitors	N06AB06	Sertraline

Figure. 8: This table illustrates the hierarchical breakdown of ATC codes for three commonly prescribed medications, demonstrating how each level progressively narrows the classification from broad anatomical group to specific chemical substance.

4.3 INTERNATIONAL CLASSIFICATION OF DISEASES (ICD)

The International Classification of Diseases (ICD) is the global standard diagnostic classification system for epidemiological purposes, health management, and clinical applications. Maintained by the World Health Organization (WHO), the ICD provides a systematic coding framework for diseases, disorders, injuries, and other health-related conditions.

The ICD serves multiple critical functions in healthcare and pharmacovigilance. It enables the systematic recording, analysis, interpretation, and comparison of mortality and morbidity data collected across different countries and time periods. In pharmacovigilance, the ICD classification is essential for coding medical history, concurrent illnesses, and adverse events, facilitating the assessment of drug-disease interactions and the identification of populations at risk.

The ICD has evolved through multiple revisions since its inception in 1893 as the International List of Causes of Death. The classification has been revised approximately every 10-15 years to incorporate new medical knowledge, changing disease patterns, and advances in medical science. Each revision expands the scope and improves the clinical utility of the classification system.

The primary purposes of the ICD include:

Statistical and epidemiological analysis: The ICD enables the collection and analysis of disease incidence and prevalence data at local, national, and international levels. This information is crucial for public health planning, resource allocation, and monitoring health trends.

Clinical documentation: Healthcare providers use ICD codes to document diagnoses, medical conditions, and reasons for healthcare encounters. This standardized documentation improves communication among healthcare professionals and supports continuity of care.

Reimbursement and insurance: Many healthcare systems use ICD codes for billing, reimbursement, and insurance claim processing, ensuring that healthcare services are appropriately documented and compensated.

Research and pharmacovigilance: The ICD provides a standardized framework for coding diseases and health conditions in clinical research, drug safety monitoring, and pharmacoepidemiological studies. In adverse drug reaction reporting, ICD codes help classify the medical events experienced by patients.

4.4 ICD-10 AND ICD-11 OVERVIEW

ICD-10 (International Classification of Diseases, 10th Revision)

ICD-10 was endorsed by the World Health Assembly in 1990 and came into use by WHO member states starting in 1994. It represents a significant expansion and reorganization compared to previous revisions, providing more detailed clinical information and accommodating new diseases and conditions.

The ICD-10 classification uses an alphanumeric coding system consisting of one letter followed by two digits at the three-character level, with optional additional characters for greater specificity. The classification is organized into 22 chapters based primarily on body systems and categories of conditions.

Structure of ICD-10 Codes:

The basic structure of ICD-10 codes consists of:

- **Category (3 characters):** Letter + two digits (e.g., I21 – Acute myocardial infarction)
- **Subcategory (4 characters):** Category + decimal point + one digit (e.g., I21.0 – Acute transmural myocardial infarction of anterior wall)
- **Further detail (5-6 characters):** Additional characters for greater specificity

ICD-10 Chapter Structure:

The 22 chapters of ICD-10 are organized as follows:

- **Chapter I (A00-B99):** Certain infectious and parasitic diseases
- **Chapter II (C00-D48):** Neoplasms
- **Chapter III (D50-D89):** Diseases of the blood and blood-forming organs
- **Chapter IV (E00-E90):** Endocrine, nutritional, and metabolic diseases
- **Chapter V (F00-F99):** Mental and behavioral disorders
- **Chapter VI (G00-G99):** Diseases of the nervous system
- **Chapter VII (H00-H59):** Diseases of the eye and adnexa
- **Chapter VIII (H60-H95):** Diseases of the ear and mastoid process

- **Chapter IX (I00-I99):** Diseases of the circulatory system
- **Chapter X (J00-J99):** Diseases of the respiratory system
- **Chapter XI (K00-K93):** Diseases of the digestive system
- **Chapter XII (L00-L99):** Diseases of the skin and subcutaneous tissue
- **Chapter XIII (M00-M99):** Diseases of the musculoskeletal system and connective tissue
- **Chapter XIV (N00-N99):** Diseases of the genitourinary system
- **Chapter XV (O00-O99):** Pregnancy, childbirth, and the puerperium
- **Chapter XVI (P00-P96):** Certain conditions originating in the perinatal period
- **Chapter XVII (Q00-Q99):** Congenital malformations and chromosomal abnormalities
- **Chapter XVIII (R00-R99):** Symptoms, signs, and abnormal findings
- **Chapter XIX (S00-T98):** Injury, poisoning, and external causes
- **Chapter XX (V01-Y98):** External causes of morbidity and mortality
- **Chapter XXI (Z00-Z99):** Factors influencing health status
- **Chapter XXII (U00-U99):** Codes for special purposes

Example of ICD-10 Coding:

Consider the ICD-10 code E11.65 (Type 2 diabetes mellitus with hyperglycemia):

- **E** – Endocrine, nutritional, and metabolic diseases
- **E11** – Type 2 diabetes mellitus

- **E11.6** – Type 2 diabetes mellitus with specified complications
- **E11.65** – Type 2 diabetes mellitus with hyperglycemia

ICD-11 (International Classification of Diseases, 11th Revision)

ICD-11 was officially adopted by the World Health Assembly in May 2019 and came into effect on January 1, 2022. This latest revision represents a fundamental transformation of the ICD, incorporating advances in medical science, digital health technology, and clinical practice.

ICD-11 introduces several major innovations:

Digital-first design: Unlike previous revisions that were primarily paper-based, ICD-11 was designed from the ground up as a digital product. The classification is fully electronic, with built-in tools for searching, browsing, and coding that improve usability and accuracy.

Enhanced clinical detail: ICD-11 provides significantly more clinical detail than ICD-10, with more than 55,000 codes compared to approximately 14,000 in ICD-10. This expanded granularity enables more precise documentation of clinical conditions.

Modernized structure: ICD-11 employs a more logical and consistent structure with improved organization of disease categories. The classification better reflects current medical knowledge and clinical practice patterns.

Multiple parenting: ICD-11 allows certain entities to appear in multiple locations within the classification hierarchy (multiple parenting), reflecting the complex nature of many medical conditions that can be classified from different perspectives.

Integration with other classifications: ICD-11 is designed to integrate seamlessly with other WHO classifications and health information standards, including ICHI (International Classification of

Health Interventions) and ICF (International Classification of Functioning, Disability, and Health).

Improved coding of traditional medicine: ICD-11 includes a supplementary chapter on traditional medicine conditions, acknowledging the importance of traditional medical systems in global healthcare.

Better representation of patient safety: The classification includes enhanced coding capabilities for adverse events, patient safety incidents, and healthcare-related harm.

Structure of ICD-11 Codes:

ICD-11 uses a combination of letters and numbers in its coding system, with a stem code providing the foundation and extension codes adding specificity. The basic structure includes:

- Stem code: Identifies the primary entity (e.g., 5A10 – Hypertensive diseases)
- Extension codes: Add clinical detail about severity, anatomy, etiology, and other dimensions

Applications in Pharmacovigilance:

Both ICD-10 and ICD-11 play crucial roles in pharmacovigilance activities:

Medical history coding: Patient medical history and pre-existing conditions are coded using ICD to assess risk factors for adverse drug reactions.

Adverse event classification: Many adverse events, particularly those manifesting as recognized disease states, are classified using ICD codes.

Comorbidity analysis: ICD codes facilitate the analysis of drug-disease interactions and the impact of comorbidities on drug safety.

Signal detection: Standardized disease coding enables the systematic identification of safety signals through statistical analysis of adverse event databases.

4.5 DEFINED DAILY DOSE (DDD)

The Defined Daily Dose (DDD) is a statistical measure of drug consumption developed by the WHO. It represents the assumed average maintenance dose per day for a drug used for its main indication in adults. The DDD provides a standardized unit of measurement that enables researchers to assess and compare drug utilization patterns across different settings, populations, and time periods.

The DDD is not necessarily the same as the recommended daily dose or the prescribed daily dose. Rather, it serves as a technical unit of measurement that remains constant regardless of variations in prescribing practices. This standardization makes the DDD particularly valuable for pharmacoepidemiological research and drug utilization studies.

Definition and Purpose:

The WHO defines the DDD as "the assumed average maintenance dose per day for a drug used for its main indication in adults." Each ATC code has an associated DDD value expressed in grams, milligrams, micrograms, international units, or other appropriate units.

The primary purposes of the DDD include:

Drug utilization comparisons: DDDs enable meaningful comparisons of drug consumption between different healthcare systems, geographic regions, or time periods, independent of variations in package sizes, formulations, or pricing.

Trend analysis: By converting drug consumption data into DDDs, researchers can track changes in prescribing patterns over time and evaluate the impact of public health interventions.

Pharmacoeconomic research: DDDs facilitate cost-effectiveness analyses by providing a standardized measure of drug exposure.

Pharmacovigilance applications: In drug safety monitoring, DDDs help estimate population exposure to medications, calculate incidence rates of adverse drug reactions, and identify changes in utilization patterns that may affect safety profiles.

Calculation and Expression:

Drug consumption data is typically converted into DDDs using the following approach:

DDD per 1000 inhabitants per day = (Total amount of drug consumed × 1000) / (DDD value × Population × Number of days)

This metric expresses how many people per 1000 in a population receive the DDD of a particular drug on an average day.

Example:

Suppose 50,000 grams of atorvastatin were consumed in a population of 100,000 people over one year. The DDD for atorvastatin (C10AA05) is 20 mg or 0.02 g.

DDD per 1000 inhabitants per day = (50,000 g × 1000) / (0.02 g × 100,000 × 365 days) = 50,000,000 / 730,000 = 68.5 DDD/1000 inhabitants/day

This indicates that approximately 68.5 people per 1000 population receive the defined daily dose of atorvastatin on an average day.

Limitations of DDD:

While the DDD is a valuable tool, it has several important limitations:

Not a recommended dose: The DDD represents an average technical measure, not a therapeutic recommendation. Actual prescribed doses may vary significantly based on patient factors and clinical indications.

Population-specific variations: The DDD is defined for adults and may not accurately reflect drug use in children, elderly patients, or other special populations.

Multiple indications: Drugs used for different indications at different doses may have only one DDD based on the main indication.

Combination products: Fixed-dose combination products require special consideration in DDD assignment and may not accurately reflect utilization of individual components.

Despite these limitations, the DDD remains an indispensable tool for drug utilization research and pharmacovigilance, providing a common language for quantifying and comparing medication use.

4.6 INTERNATIONAL NON-PROPRIETARY NAMES (INN) FOR DRUGS

International Non-proprietary Names (INN) are unique, globally recognized names for pharmaceutical substances established by the World Health Organization. INNs provide a universal nomenclature system that facilitates clear communication about medicines across linguistic, cultural, and national boundaries.

The concept of INN was developed to address the confusion arising from multiple brand names, trade names, and local names for the same pharmaceutical substance. By providing a single, standardized name for each active substance, the INN system enhances patient safety, supports rational prescribing, enables effective pharmacovigilance, and facilitates international collaboration in drug regulation and research.

Purpose and Importance:

The INN system serves several critical functions:

Patient safety: Using standardized INNs reduces medication errors caused by confusion between different brand names for the same active substance or similar names for different substances.

Global communication: INNs enable healthcare professionals, regulators, and researchers worldwide to communicate unambiguously about pharmaceutical substances.

Pharmacovigilance: Standardized naming is essential for adverse drug reaction reporting, signal detection, and safety database management. INN ensures that reports about the same substance from different countries can be properly aggregated and analyzed.

Prescribing and dispensing: Many countries mandate or encourage prescribing by INN rather than brand name to promote rational drug use and facilitate generic substitution.

Regulatory harmonization: INNs support international regulatory cooperation by providing a common reference point for drug approval, labeling, and post-marketing surveillance.

Principles of INN Selection:

The selection of INNs follows specific linguistic and scientific principles:

Distinctiveness: INNs should be distinctive in sound and spelling to minimize confusion with existing INNs and avoid medication errors.

Commonality: Related substances with similar pharmacological properties often share common stems (affixes) that indicate their therapeutic class.

Simplicity: INNs should be relatively short, easy to pronounce in major languages, and suitable for use as brand names in various linguistic contexts.

No commercial implications: INNs should not suggest commercial advantage or convey promotional messages about the substance.

Common Stems in INN:

The INN system employs common stems (prefixes, infixes, or suffixes) to group substances with related structure or pharmacological action. Recognizing these stems helps healthcare professionals and pharmacovigilance specialists identify the therapeutic class of unfamiliar substances.

Table 9: Common INN Stems and Their Meanings

Stem	Position	Therapeutic Class	Examples
-azepam	Suffix	Benzodiazepines (diazepam type)	Diazepam, Lorazepam, Alprazolam
-olol	Suffix	Beta-blockers	Propranolol, Atenolol, Metoprolol
-pril	Suffix	ACE inhibitors	Enalapril, Lisinopril, Ramipril
-sartan	Suffix	Angiotensin II receptor antagonists	Losartan, Valsartan, Telmisartan
-statin	Suffix	HMG-CoA reductase inhibitors	Atorvastatin, Simvastatin, Rosuvastatin
-cillin	Suffix	Penicillin-type antibiotics	Penicillin, Ampicillin, Amoxicillin
Cef-	Prefix	Cephalosporin antibiotics	Cefuroxime, Ceftriaxone, Cefixime
-coxib	Suffix	COX-2 inhibitors	Celecoxib, Etoricoxib, Parecoxib
-mycin	Suffix	Macrolide antibiotics	Erythromycin, Azithromycin, Clarithromycin
-triptan	Suffix	5-HT_1 agonists (antimigraine)	Sumatriptan, Rizatriptan, Zolmitriptan

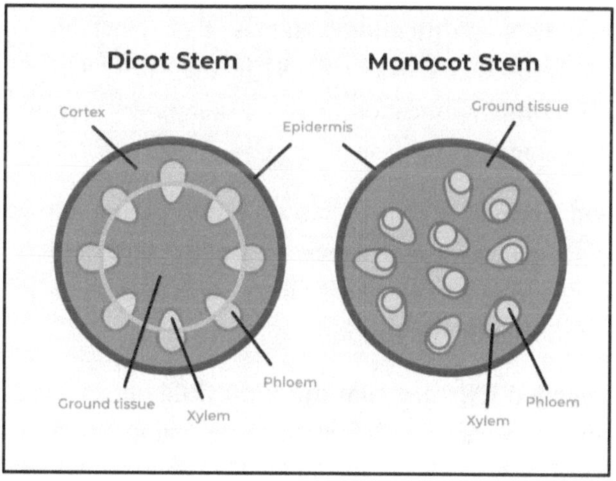

Figure 9: This table presents frequently encountered INN stems that indicate specific therapeutic classes.

4.7 WHO INN PROGRAMME

The WHO INN Programme is responsible for selecting, developing, and disseminating International Non-proprietary Names for pharmaceutical substances. Established in 1950, the programme operates under the authority of the World Health Assembly and coordinates with national nomenclature authorities, pharmaceutical manufacturers, and regulatory agencies worldwide.

Structure and Process:

The INN Programme follows a systematic procedure for reviewing and selecting names for new pharmaceutical substances:

Submission: Pharmaceutical manufacturers or other interested parties submit proposals for INNs for new substances during drug development, typically before or during clinical trials.

Technical review: The WHO INN Expert Group evaluates proposed names according to established criteria, checking for distinctiveness, appropriate use of stems, pronunciation across languages, and potential for confusion with existing names.

Proposed INN publication: Names that meet the criteria are published as "proposed INNs" (pINN) in the WHO Drug Information bulletin. During this publication phase, stakeholders worldwide have an opportunity to comment or raise objections.

Objection period: A four-month objection period allows healthcare professionals, regulatory authorities, and other stakeholders to identify potential problems with proposed names, such as similarity to existing names or pronunciation difficulties.

Recommended INN designation: If no valid objections are received, or after any necessary modifications, the name is designated as a "recommended INN" (rINN) and published in subsequent WHO Drug Information bulletins and cumulative lists.

INN Database and Publications:

The WHO maintains comprehensive resources documenting all designated INNs:

INN database: An online, searchable database containing all proposed and recommended INNs, including chemical structures, molecular formulas, and assigned ATC codes.

WHO Drug Information: A quarterly bulletin that publishes newly proposed and recommended INNs, along with technical information and updates to the programme.

Cumulative lists: Periodically updated compilations of all recommended INNs, organized alphabetically and by therapeutic class.

These resources serve as authoritative references for healthcare professionals, regulators, and researchers worldwide, supporting accurate drug identification and communication.

Modified INN (INNM):

For substances that are salts, esters, or derivatives of a parent compound, the WHO uses modified INNs (INNMs). The INNM consists of the parent INN plus a modifier indicating the specific salt or ester form. For example:

- Metoprolol (parent INN)
- Metoprolol tartrate (INNM)
- Metoprolol succinate (INNM)

This system maintains the recognition of the parent compound while clearly distinguishing different forms that may have distinct pharmaceutical properties.

National Nomenclature Coordination:

Many countries have established national nomenclature authorities that coordinate with the WHO INN Programme. These national bodies may adopt INNs as official names in their countries, adapt INN stems for local linguistic requirements, or maintain parallel national naming systems. Close coordination between the WHO and national authorities ensures global consistency while accommodating local needs.

The United States Adopted Names (USAN) Council, the British Pharmacopoeia Commission, the Japanese Adopted Names (JAN) Programme, and similar bodies in other countries work collaboratively with WHO to harmonize nomenclature and minimize discrepancies between international and national names.

INN in Pharmacovigilance Practice:

In pharmacovigilance, the use of INNs is fundamental to accurate adverse event reporting and data management:

Case report forms: International Council for Harmonisation (ICH) guidelines recommend reporting suspected drugs in individual case safety reports using INNs to ensure global interpretability.

Database coding: Pharmacovigilance databases use INNs as the primary identifier for active substances, linking brand names and local names to the corresponding INN for standardized analysis.

Signal detection: Aggregating adverse event reports by INN enables the identification of safety signals that might be obscured if reports were fragmented across multiple brand names.

Literature surveillance: Pharmacovigilance teams conducting literature searches use INNs to comprehensively identify relevant safety information regardless of the brand names mentioned in publications.

This chapter has provided a comprehensive overview of the fundamental classification and nomenclature systems that underpin modern pharmacovigilance practice. The Anatomical Therapeutic Chemical (ATC) classification system offers a robust, hierarchical framework for organizing pharmaceutical substances based on their anatomical target, therapeutic purpose, and chemical properties. Its five-level structure enables both broad categorical analysis and precise substance identification, making it indispensable for drug utilization research and pharmacovigilance activities.

The International Classification of Diseases (ICD), particularly the current ICD-10 and emerging ICD-11 systems, provides the global standard for coding diseases, injuries, and health conditions. These classification systems enable standardized documentation of medical history, concurrent illnesses, and adverse events, facilitating meaningful comparisons across healthcare settings and supporting evidence-based safety assessments.

The Defined Daily Dose (DDD) concept offers a standardized metric for quantifying and comparing drug consumption, enabling researchers to track utilization patterns and estimate population exposure to medications. While the DDD has limitations and must be interpreted carefully, it remains an essential tool for pharmacoepidemiological research and drug safety monitoring.

International Non-proprietary Names (INN) provide the linguistic foundation for global pharmacovigilance, ensuring that healthcare professionals, regulators, and researchers worldwide can communicate unambiguously about pharmaceutical substances. The WHO INN Programme's systematic approach to selecting and disseminating standardized names enhances patient safety, supports rational prescribing, and facilitates international regulatory cooperation.

Together, these classification and nomenclature systems form the common language of pharmacovigilance. Mastery of these systems is essential for students and practitioners who will contribute to drug safety monitoring in hospitals, regulatory agencies, pharmaceutical companies, and international organizations. The standardized frameworks described in this chapter enable the aggregation, analysis, and interpretation of safety data from diverse sources, ultimately supporting the goal of protecting public health through vigilant monitoring of medicinal products.

CHAPTER 5

DRUG DICTIONARIES AND CODING IN PHARMACOVIGILANCE

KEY OUTCOMES

Upon completion of this chapter, learners will be able to:

1. Understand the historical development and structure of WHO Adverse Reaction Terminology (WHO-ART)
2. Explain the comprehensive structure of the Medical Dictionary for Regulatory Activities (MedDRA)
3. Describe the five-level MedDRA hierarchy and its application in adverse event coding
4. Define Standardised MedDRA Queries (SMQs) and their role in safety signal detection
5. Understand the structure and function of the WHO Drug Dictionary
6. Explain principles of drug coding and substance identification in pharmacovigilance
7. Describe the EudraVigilance Medicinal Product Dictionary and its regulatory applications
8. Apply standardized terminologies for accurate adverse event and product coding

ABSTRACT

Standardized medical and drug terminology is the cornerstone of effective pharmacovigilance. This chapter examines the principal terminologies and dictionaries used for coding adverse events and medicinal products in drug safety reporting. The Medical Dictionary for Regulatory Activities (MedDRA) provides an internationally standardized terminology for coding adverse events, medical history, and indications in regulatory submissions. The WHO Adverse Reaction Terminology (WHO-ART), though largely superseded by MedDRA, played a historical role in establishing standardized adverse event coding. Drug dictionaries, including the WHO Drug Dictionary and EudraVigilance Medicinal Product Dictionary, enable precise identification and coding of medicinal products involved in adverse events. Understanding these terminologies and their hierarchical structures is essential for accurate data entry, retrieval, signal detection, and regulatory reporting in pharmacovigilance. This chapter systematically presents the structure, application, and practical utilization of these standardized terminologies in contemporary drug safety practice.

5.1 WHO ADVERSE REACTION TERMINOLOGY (WHO-ART)

The **WHO Adverse Reaction Terminology (WHO-ART)** was one of the first internationally recognized standardized terminologies developed specifically for coding adverse drug reactions in pharmacovigilance. Developed by the Uppsala Monitoring Centre (UMC), which serves as the WHO Collaborating Centre for International Drug Monitoring, WHO-ART was widely used in the WHO Programme for International Drug Monitoring from 1971 until it was gradually replaced by MedDRA in the early 2000s.

Historical Context and Purpose:

WHO-ART was created to address the need for consistent terminology in the WHO's global database of adverse drug reaction reports. Before standardized terminologies existed, different countries and organizations used different terms to describe the same adverse events, making it difficult to aggregate and analyze safety data internationally. WHO-ART provided a common language that enabled meaningful comparisons of adverse reaction patterns across countries and facilitated the early detection of drug safety signals.

The terminology was specifically designed for pharmacovigilance rather than general medical coding, focusing on terms commonly used to describe adverse drug reactions, poisonings, and drug-related medical events. This targeted approach made WHO-ART particularly well-suited for spontaneous reporting systems, where the primary concern is capturing drug safety information rather than comprehensive medical diagnosis.

Structure of WHO-ART:

WHO-ART employed a hierarchical four-level structure that organized adverse reaction terms from general to specific:

Level 1 - System Organ Class (SOC): The highest level categorized adverse reactions according to the body system affected or the etiology of the reaction. WHO-ART included 33 System Organ Classes covering major organ systems and categories of disorders.

Examples of SOCs included:

- Cardiovascular disorders
- Gastrointestinal system disorders
- Nervous system disorders
- Skin and appendages disorders
- Respiratory system disorders
- Body as a whole - general disorders

Level 2 - High Level Terms: These provided a therapeutic or anatomical subgrouping within each SOC, offering intermediate specificity between the broad SOC and specific preferred terms.

Level 3 - Preferred Terms (PTs): This was the primary working level of WHO-ART, containing specific medical terms used to code individual adverse reactions. Each preferred term represented a distinct medical concept or symptom.

Level 4 - Included Terms: The lowest level contained synonyms, colloquialisms, and alternative expressions that mapped to the corresponding preferred term. This level facilitated data entry by allowing reporters to use various terms while ensuring standardized coding.

Example of WHO-ART Hierarchy:

Consider the adverse reaction "myocardial infarction":

- **SOC:** Cardiovascular disorders
- **High Level Term:** Heart rate and rhythm disorders
- **Preferred Term:** Myocardial infarction
- **Included Terms:** Heart attack, MI, acute MI, coronary thrombosis

Limitations and Transition to MedDRA:

While WHO-ART served pharmacovigilance well for several decades, it had limitations that became increasingly apparent:

Limited scope: WHO-ART contained approximately 1,800 preferred terms, which proved insufficient for coding the full spectrum of adverse events reported in modern pharmacovigilance.

Infrequent updates: The terminology was updated relatively infrequently, making it difficult to incorporate new medical concepts and emerging adverse reactions.

Lack of multiaxiality: Each preferred term belonged to only one SOC, which did not reflect the reality that some adverse events could logically be classified under multiple organ systems.

Limited granularity: The terminology lacked the detailed specificity needed for coding complex adverse events and distinguishing between closely related conditions.

These limitations led to the development of MedDRA, which addressed these shortcomings while retaining compatibility with WHO-ART to facilitate data migration. Although WHO-ART is no longer actively maintained, understanding its structure remains valuable for historical pharmacovigilance data analysis and for appreciating the evolution of medical terminology in drug safety monitoring.

5.2 MEDICAL DICTIONARY FOR REGULATORY ACTIVITIES (MedDRA)

The **Medical Dictionary for Regulatory Activities (MedDRA)** is the current international medical terminology standard used for regulatory communication and evaluation of data pertaining to medicinal products. Developed under the auspices of the International Council for Harmonisation of Technical Requirements for Pharmaceuticals for Human Use (ICH), MedDRA provides a comprehensive, clinically validated terminology for coding adverse events, medical history, indications, and other medically relevant information in regulatory submissions.

Development and Governance:

MedDRA was developed in the 1990s through a collaborative effort involving regulatory authorities and the pharmaceutical industry from the ICH regions (Europe, United States, and Japan). The project began in 1994, and the first version of MedDRA was released in 1999. The terminology was designed to overcome the limitations of existing terminologies and provide a single standard that could be used across all phases of drug development and throughout the product lifecycle.

The **Maintenance and Support Services Organization (MSSO)**, operated under contract to ICH, is responsible for maintaining, updating, and distributing MedDRA. The MSSO coordinates with the **Medical Dictionary for Regulatory Activities Management Committee (MMC)**, which provides strategic oversight and direction for the terminology's development.

Purpose and Applications:

MedDRA serves multiple critical functions in pharmaceutical regulation and pharmacovigilance:

Regulatory submissions: MedDRA is the required terminology for coding adverse events in Individual Case Safety Reports (ICSRs), Periodic Benefit-Risk Evaluation Reports (PBRERs), and clinical trial submissions to regulatory authorities worldwide.

Signal detection: The standardized structure of MedDRA enables systematic statistical analysis of adverse event databases to identify potential safety signals.

Data exchange: MedDRA facilitates the electronic exchange of safety information between pharmaceutical companies, regulatory authorities, and international drug monitoring organizations.

Aggregate reporting: The hierarchical structure supports aggregation and analysis of adverse event data at various levels of specificity, from broad organ system effects to specific medical events.

Clinical trial reporting: MedDRA is used throughout clinical development to code adverse events, medical history, primary diagnoses, and secondary diagnoses in case report forms.

Post-marketing surveillance: Spontaneous reporting systems, registries, and observational studies use MedDRA to standardize adverse event documentation.

Linguistic Coverage:

One of MedDRA's significant advantages is its availability in multiple languages, facilitating its use in global drug development and pharmacovigilance. MedDRA is officially available in English, Japanese, Chinese, French, German, Spanish, Portuguese, Italian, Czech, Dutch, and Hungarian, with translations maintained by the MSSO to ensure terminological consistency across languages.

5.3 MedDRA HIERARCHY AND STRUCTURE

MedDRA employs a sophisticated **five-level hierarchical structure** that enables coding and retrieval of medical information at varying levels of specificity. Unlike WHO-ART's single path hierarchy, MedDRA's multiaxial structure allows terms to be linked to multiple System Organ Classes, reflecting the complex reality of medical events that may affect multiple body systems.

Level 1: System Organ Classes (SOCs)

The highest level of the MedDRA hierarchy consists of **26 System Organ Classes** that represent broad physiological, pathological, or etiological categories. SOCs are used for the broadest level of analysis and reporting, such as in summary tabulations of clinical trial safety data.

The 26 MedDRA SOCs are:

1. Blood and lymphatic system disorders
2. Cardiac disorders
3. Congenital, familial and genetic disorders
4. Ear and labyrinth disorders
5. Endocrine disorders
6. Eye disorders

7. Gastrointestinal disorders
8. General disorders and administration site conditions
9. Hepatobiliary disorders
10. Immune system disorders
11. Infections and infestations
12. Injury, poisoning and procedural complications
13. Investigations (laboratory and diagnostic findings)
14. Metabolism and nutrition disorders
15. Musculoskeletal and connective tissue disorders
16. Neoplasms benign, malignant and unspecified
17. Nervous system disorders
18. Pregnancy, puerperium and perinatal conditions
19. Product issues (problems with the physical product)
20. Psychiatric disorders
21. Renal and urinary disorders
22. Reproductive system and breast disorders
23. Respiratory, thoracic and mediastinal disorders
24. Skin and subcutaneous tissue disorders
25. Social circumstances
26. Surgical and medical procedures

Level 2: High Level Group Terms (HLGTs)

High Level Group Terms provide superordinate groupings of related High-Level Terms within each SOC. MedDRA contains approximately

335 HLGTs that offer an intermediate level of categorization between SOCs and HLTs.

Example within Cardiac disorders SOC:

- Cardiac arrhythmias
- Coronary artery disorders
- Heart failures

Level 3: High Level Terms (HLTs)

High Level Terms represent a level of clinical or pathophysiological specificity within each HLGT. There are approximately 1,720 HLTs in MedDRA, providing a useful level of aggregation for many analytical purposes.

Example within Cardiac arrhythmias HLGT:

- Supraventricular arrhythmias
- Ventricular arrhythmias and cardiac arrest
- Arrhythmias not specified as atrial or ventricular

Level 4: Preferred Terms (PTs)

Preferred Terms are the key working level of MedDRA, representing distinct medical concepts or conditions. MedDRA contains approximately 24,000 PTs. Each adverse event should be coded to exactly one PT, which is the most specific term that accurately describes the event.

PTs represent:

- Signs and symptoms (e.g., Headache, Nausea)
- Diseases and diagnoses (e.g., Myocardial infarction, Pneumonia)
- Investigations and their qualitative results (e.g., Blood pressure increased)

- Surgical and medical procedures (e.g., Appendicectomy)
- Medical, social, and family history findings (e.g., Hypertension, Alcohol abuse)
- Example within Supraventricular arrhythmias HLT:
- Atrial fibrillation
- Atrial flutter
- Supraventricular tachycardia

Level 5: Lowest Level Terms (LLTs)

Lowest Level Terms are the entry level of MedDRA, containing approximately 84,000 terms that represent how information may be communicated in practice. LLTs include current medical terminology, synonyms, lexical variants, quasi-synonyms, and sometimes outdated terminology that may still appear in medical records or reports.

Multiple LLTs link to each PT, enabling data entry personnel to select appropriate terminology while ensuring standardized coding. The system automatically maps the selected LLT to its corresponding PT for data analysis.

Example LLTs mapping to the PT "Myocardial infarction":

- Myocardial infarction
- Heart attack
- MI
- Acute myocardial infarction
- AMI
- Coronary thrombosis
- Cardiac infarction

Table 10: Example of Complete MedDRA Hierarchy

Level	Term Type	Example
1	SOC	Cardiac disorders
2	HLGT	Cardiac arrhythmias
3	HLT	Supraventricular arrhythmias
4	PT	Atrial fibrillation
5	LLT	Atrial fibrillation, Auricular fibrillation, AF, AFib, Atrial fibrillation NOS

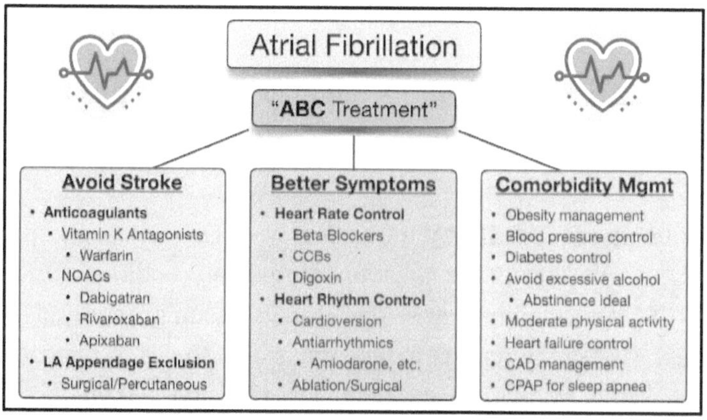

Figure 10: This table illustrates the complete five-level MedDRA hierarchy for the adverse event of atrial fibrillation, demonstrating how the structure progresses from broad organ system classification to specific preferred term and multiple entry-level synonyms.

Multiaxiality:

A critical feature of MedDRA is its **multiaxial** structure, meaning that a single PT may be linked to multiple SOCs through different pathways. This reflects clinical reality, where a medical event may appropriately be classified from multiple perspectives.

For example, the PT "Hepatic failure" appears in:

- **Primary SOC:** Hepatobiliary disorders
- **Secondary SOC:** Investigations (when reported as a laboratory finding)

This multiaxiality enables flexible retrieval and analysis while maintaining standardized coding at the PT level.

Primary and Secondary Paths:

When a PT is linked to multiple SOCs, one pathway is designated as the **primary path**, and others are **secondary paths**. The primary path generally represents the most clinically intuitive or commonly used classification. For routine reporting and tabulation, the primary SOC is typically used, but secondary paths enable alternative analyses when needed.

5.4 STANDARDISED MedDRA QUERIES (SMQs)

Standardised MedDRA Queries (SMQs) are groupings of MedDRA terms that relate to defined medical conditions or areas of interest. SMQs facilitate the retrieval, screening, and analysis of individual case safety reports for specific safety topics, supporting signal detection, safety evaluation, and regulatory decision-making.

Purpose and Development:

SMQs were developed to address the challenge of comprehensively identifying all cases relevant to a particular medical condition of interest. When searching for adverse events related to conditions like hepatotoxicity or rhabdomyolysis, it is not sufficient to search for a single preferred term. A comprehensive search must include related signs, symptoms, laboratory abnormalities, diagnostic terms, and procedures.

SMQs provide pre-validated groupings of relevant MedDRA terms for important safety topics, eliminating the need for each organization to independently develop search strategies. This standardization improves the consistency, efficiency, and comparability of safety analyses across organizations and studies.

SMQs are developed through a rigorous process involving:

- Expert clinical input from subject matter specialists
- Review and validation by regulatory authorities
- Testing with real-world adverse event data
- Periodic updates to incorporate new terms and refine scope

Types of SMQs:

SMQs are classified into several categories based on their medical focus:

Organ-specific SMQs: Focus on conditions affecting specific organ systems (e.g., Acute renal failure, Liver injury)

Pathophysiological SMQs: Address specific pathophysiological mechanisms (e.g., Anaphylactic reactions, Rhabdomyolysis)

Etiology-based SMQs: Group events by causative mechanism (e.g., Drug-induced liver injury)

Demographic SMQs: Focus on conditions affecting specific populations (e.g., Pregnancy and neonatal topics)

Structure of SMQs:

Each SMQ consists of a defined list of MedDRA Preferred Terms (PTs) selected to comprehensively represent the medical condition of interest. SMQs are organized into **narrow** and **broad** scope levels:

Narrow scope: Contains PTs that are highly specific for the condition, with a high likelihood that the reported event represents the condition of interest. Narrow searches prioritize specificity over sensitivity, minimizing false positives.

Broad scope: Includes all narrow scope terms plus additional PTs that may represent the condition but could also indicate other diagnoses. Broad searches prioritize sensitivity, ensuring comprehensive case identification at the cost of including some false positives.

Example: SMQ for Hepatic Disorders

The Hepatic disorders SMQ (narrow scope) might include highly specific terms such as:

- Hepatic failure
- Drug-induced liver injury
- Hepatocellular injury
- Acute hepatic failure

The broad scope would additionally include less specific terms like:

- Hepatic enzyme increased
- Liver function test abnormal
- Jaundice
- Hepatomegaly

Applications of SMQs:

SMQs support multiple pharmacovigilance activities:

Signal detection: SMQs enable systematic screening of adverse event databases for specific safety concerns, identifying potential signals that might be missed with simple term searches.

Periodic safety reporting: Pharmaceutical companies use SMQs to identify relevant cases for inclusion in Periodic Safety Update Reports (PSURs) and Periodic Benefit-Risk Evaluation Reports (PBRERs).

Safety assessments: Regulatory authorities and pharmaceutical companies use SMQs to conduct focused safety evaluations in response to emerging safety concerns.

Clinical trial monitoring: SMQs facilitate real-time monitoring of adverse events of special interest during clinical trials, supporting data monitoring committee activities.

Risk management: SMQs help identify cases for inclusion in risk management plan activities and evaluation of risk minimization measure effectiveness.

Currently Available SMQs:

As of recent releases, MedDRA includes over 100 SMQs covering a wide range of important safety topics, including:

- Acute pancreatitis
- Anaphylactic reaction
- Angioedema
- Cardiac arrhythmias
- Drug abuse, dependence and withdrawal
- Embolic and thrombotic events
- Haemorrhage terms (excluding laboratory terms)
- Interstitial lung disease
- Malignancies
- Pregnancy and neonatal topics
- Rhabdomyolysis/myopathy
- Severe cutaneous adverse reactions

The SMQ list is continuously expanded and refined based on regulatory and industry needs, emerging safety concerns, and advances in medical understandin.

5.5 WHO DRUG DICTIONARY

The **WHO Drug Dictionary** is a comprehensive database of medicinal product information maintained by the Uppsala Monitoring Centre for use in international drug safety monitoring. It serves as the primary reference for coding medicinal products in the WHO global database of individual case safety reports (VigiBase) and is widely used by regulatory authorities, pharmaceutical companies, and research organizations worldwide.

Purpose and Content:

The WHO Drug Dictionary provides standardized identification and coding of medicinal products involved in adverse drug reaction reports. The dictionary enables:

Substance identification: Linking reported drugs to their active pharmaceutical ingredients using International Non-proprietary Names (INN)

Product standardization: Associating trade names, brand names, and local product names with standardized substance and product records

ATC classification: Providing ATC codes for substances to facilitate therapeutic class analysis

Formulation information: Including dosage forms, strengths, and routes of administration

International coverage: Encompassing products from over 150 countries with both proprietary and non-proprietary names

Structure and Components:

The WHO Drug Dictionary is organized around several key data elements:

Medicinal Product: The specific proprietary or trade name of the product as marketed (e.g., Lipitor, Zocor)

Active Substance: The pharmacologically active ingredient(s) using INN terminology (e.g., atorvastatin, simvastatin)

ATC Code: The assigned Anatomical Therapeutic Chemical classification code

Dosage Form: The pharmaceutical formulation (e.g., tablet, capsule, injection)

Strength: The concentration or amount of active substance

Route of Administration: The pathway by which the drug is administered (e.g., oral, intravenous, topical)

Manufacturer/License Holder: The company responsible for marketing the product

Country: The country or region where the product is marketed

Coding Principles:

When coding medicinal products in adverse drug reaction reports using the WHO Drug Dictionary, several principles apply:

Substance-based coding: The primary focus is on identifying the active pharmaceutical ingredient(s) rather than the specific brand, supporting analysis by active substance across different marketed products.

Combination products: Fixed-dose combination products are coded to indicate all active ingredients, enabling analysis of both individual components and the combination.

Specificity: The most specific product information available should be captured, including dosage form and strength when known.

Standardization: Local or colloquial drug names should be linked to standardized INN names for international comparability.

5.6 DRUG CODING AND SUBSTANCE IDENTIFICATION

Drug coding in pharmacovigilance refers to the systematic process of identifying and standardizing information about medicinal products reported in adverse event cases. Accurate drug coding is essential for retrieving cases, conducting signal detection, and ensuring regulatory compliance. The process involves linking the reported drug name (which may be a brand name, generic name, or local name) to standardized substance and product records in drug dictionaries.

Steps in Drug Coding:

The drug coding process typically follows these steps:

Data capture: Recording drug information from the adverse event report, including product name, active ingredients, dosage form, strength, route of administration, and manufacturer.

Dictionary search: Searching the drug dictionary (WHO Drug Dictionary, EudraVigilance dictionary, or proprietary databases) using the reported product name or active ingredient.

Product selection: Selecting the appropriate dictionary record that matches the reported product, considering factors such as geographic availability, formulation, and manufacturer.

Substance identification: Linking the product to its active pharmaceutical ingredient(s) using standardized INN nomenclature.

ATC classification: Assigning the appropriate ATC code(s) for the active substance(s).

Quality check: Verifying that the selected code accurately represents the reported drug and that all relevant fields are completed.

Challenges in Drug Coding:

Several challenges commonly arise in drug coding:

Incomplete information: Reporters may provide incomplete drug information, such as brand names without dosage forms or generic names without specifying the salt form.

Multiple names: The same active substance may be marketed under numerous brand names in different countries, requiring extensive cross-referencing.

Combination products: Fixed-dose combinations require coding of all active ingredients and recognition of the specific combination product.

Local variations: Local or regional drug names, particularly in non-English speaking countries, may not be readily identifiable in international dictionaries.

Novel products: New products may not yet be included in drug dictionaries, requiring special handling and dictionary updates.

Herbal and traditional medicines: Products containing multiple plant extracts or traditional medicine ingredients pose coding challenges due to variable composition and limited standardization.

Substance Identification Best Practices:

To ensure accurate substance identification:

Use INN names: Always link products to their INN names for international standardization.

Specify salt forms: When relevant, distinguish between different salt forms of the same base substance (e.g., metoprolol tartrate vs. metoprolol succinate).

Code all active ingredients: For combination products, ensure all active components are coded.

Document verbatim: Retain the verbatim drug name as reported alongside the coded standardized name.

Verify geographic availability: Confirm that the selected product is marketed in the country of the reporter.

Update regularly: Use the most current version of drug dictionaries to access the latest product information and newly registered substances.

5.7 EUDRAVIGILANCE MEDICINAL PRODUCT DICTIONARY

The **EudraVigilance Medicinal Product Dictionary (EVMPD)** is the European Medicines Agency's reference database for identifying and describing medicinal products authorized in the European Economic Area (EEA). It serves as the standard for coding medicinal products in the EudraVigilance database, which collects and analyzes Individual Case Safety Reports submitted to the European regulatory network.

Purpose and Scope:

EVMPD provides comprehensive information about authorized medicinal products including active substances, proprietary names, pharmaceutical forms, routes of administration, marketing authorization holders, and authorization status. The dictionary covers products authorized through centralized, mutual recognition, decentralized, and national procedures within the EEA.

Key Data Elements:

The EVMPD contains several essential data components:

Medicinal Product ID: Unique identifier for each authorized product **Active Substance**: INN or common name of the active ingredient **Product Name**: Trade or proprietary name **Pharmaceutical Form**:

Formulation type (tablet, solution, etc.) **Authorization Number**: Regulatory approval reference **Marketing Authorization Holder**: Company responsible for the product **ATC Code**: Therapeutic classification **Authorization Status**: Current regulatory status.

Integration with Regulatory Reporting:

Marketing authorization holders and regulatory authorities use EVMPD when submitting ICSRs to EudraVigilance. The dictionary ensures that product identification is standardized across all reports, facilitating signal detection and regulatory assessment. Companies must code suspected and concomitant medicinal products using EVMPD identifiers in their electronic submissions.

5.8 PRODUCT CODING IN PHARMACOVIGILANCE

Product coding extends beyond simple substance identification to include comprehensive documentation of the specific medicinal product involved in an adverse event. This includes formulation details, dosage regimen, indication, and temporal relationship to the event.

Essential Product Information:

Complete product coding requires capturing:

Product identification: Brand name, generic name, and dictionary code **Formulation details**: Dosage form, strength, and route of administration **Dosage regimen**: Dose, frequency, and duration of use **Indication**: Reason for use (coded using MedDRA) **Action taken**: Whether the drug was continued, discontinued, or dose modified **Rechallenge information**: Whether the patient was re-exposed to thc drug and the outcome **Concomitant medications**: Other drugs taken concurrently.

Role of Product Coding:

Accurate product coding supports multiple pharmacovigilance functions:

Case assessment: Enables evaluation of temporal relationship and biological plausibility **Signal detection**: Facilitates identification of product-specific versus class-wide safety issues **Regulatory compliance**: Ensures submissions meet regulatory requirements for product identification **Data retrieval**: Allows efficient searching and filtering of safety databases **Duplicate detection**: Helps identify duplicate reports of the same case.

Quality Assurance:

Product coding quality is maintained through:

- Use of standardized dictionaries and coding guidelines
- Regular training of coding personnel
- Automated validation checks during data entry
- Periodic audits of coded data
- Resolution of coding queries and inconsistencies

Proper product coding ensures that pharmacovigilance databases contain accurate, retrievable, and analyzable information essential for protecting public health through effective drug safety monitoring.

Standardised MedDRA Queries (SMQs) represent an important advancement in pharmacovigilance methodology, enabling consistent and comprehensive case identification for important safety topics. Drug dictionaries, including the WHO Drug Dictionary and EudraVigilance Medicinal Product Dictionary, provide the essential infrastructure for standardized product identification and coding.

CHAPTER 6

INFORMATION RESOURCES IN PHARMACOVIGILANCE

KEY OUTCOMES

Upon completion of this chapter, learners will be able to:

1. Identify and describe basic drug information resources used in pharmacovigilance
2. Understand the role and content of pharmacopoeias as official drug standards
3. Explain the purpose and application of drug compendia and formularies
4. Describe specialized resources for adverse drug reactions and their use in safety assessment
5. Understand the structure and content of Micromedex and Drugdex systems
6. Explain the role of the WHO Pharmaceuticals Newsletter in global safety communication
7. Describe FDA MedWatch and its function in drug safety reporting
8. Identify key electronic databases for pharmacovigilance literature surveillance

ABSTRACT

Effective pharmacovigilance practice requires access to reliable, comprehensive, and current information resources about drugs, adverse reactions, and drug safety. This chapter examines the principal information resources used in pharmacovigilance activities, ranging from basic reference materials to specialized databases and electronic resources. Pharmacopoeias provide official standards for drug quality and composition. Drug compendia and formularies offer comprehensive prescribing information and therapeutic guidance. Specialized resources such as Micromedex and Drugdex provide evidence-based information specifically focused on adverse drug reactions, drug interactions, and toxicology. Regulatory publications like the WHO Pharmaceuticals Newsletter and FDA MedWatch provide timely safety alerts and regulatory actions. Electronic databases enable systematic literature surveillance and signal detection. Understanding the scope, content, and appropriate application of these diverse resources is essential for conducting thorough pharmacovigilance assessments and making evidence-based decisions in drug safety practice.

6.1 BASIC DRUG INFORMATION RESOURCES

Basic drug information resources provide fundamental information about medicinal products including indications, dosing, contraindications, warnings, adverse reactions, and drug interactions. These resources serve as the first reference point for pharmacovigilance professionals conducting case assessment, literature review, and safety evaluation.

Categories of Basic Resources:

Product information documents: Package inserts, Summary of Product Characteristics (SmPC), and prescribing information approved by regulatory authorities provide the official, legally binding information about a medicinal product.

Reference textbooks: Comprehensive pharmacology and therapeutics textbooks provide detailed information about drug classes, mechanisms of action, pharmacokinetics, and clinical applications.

Drug handbooks: Portable references designed for quick consultation, containing essential prescribing information in condensed format.

Online databases: Web-based resources providing searchable drug information with regular updates and links to primary literature.

Key Basic Resources:

Martindale: The Complete Drug Reference provides comprehensive information on drugs and medicines used worldwide, including synonyms, chemical properties, adverse effects, precautions, interactions, and therapeutic uses.

British National Formulary (BNF) offers practical prescribing information for healthcare professionals in the United Kingdom, with detailed guidance on drug selection, dosing, and safety.

American Hospital Formulary Service Drug Information (AHFS-DI) provides evidence-based, peer-reviewed drug information organized by therapeutic class.

Drug Facts and Comparisons present comparative information on therapeutic drug classes, facilitating evidence-based drug selection.

Physicians' Desk Reference (PDR) compiles FDA-approved product labeling for prescription drugs marketed in the United States.

Applications in Pharmacovigilance:

These basic resources support pharmacovigilance activities by:

- Providing reference information for case assessment and causality evaluation
- Identifying known adverse reactions and risk factors
- Verifying appropriate indications and dosing
- Documenting baseline safety information for signal evaluation
- Supporting medical review and quality assurance activities

6.2 PHARMACOPOEIAS

Pharmacopoeias are official compendia that establish legally recognized standards for the identity, strength, quality, purity, and preparation of medicines. While primarily focused on pharmaceutical quality rather than clinical use, pharmacopoeias provide authoritative reference information relevant to drug safety assessment.

Major International Pharmacopoeias:

United States Pharmacopeia (USP) and National Formulary (NF) establish quality standards for medicines, dietary supplements, and food ingredients marketed in the United States.

European Pharmacopoeia (Ph. Eur.) provides harmonized quality standards for medicines used in European countries, maintained by the European Directorate for the Quality of Medicines.

British Pharmacopoeia (BP) contains standards for medicinal substances and formulations used in the United Kingdom.

International Pharmacopoeia (Ph.Int.) published by WHO provides internationally applicable standards, particularly valuable for countries without national pharmacopoeias.

Indian Pharmacopoeia (IP) establishes official standards for drugs manufactured and marketed in India.

Japanese Pharmacopoeia (JP) provides quality standards for pharmaceuticals in Japan.

Content and Organization:

Pharmacopoeias typically contain:

Monographs: Detailed specifications for individual drugs including chemical structure, identification tests, purity requirements, and assay methods.

General chapters: Methodologies, procedures, and requirements applicable to multiple drugs.

Excipient standards: Specifications for inactive ingredients used in formulations.

Dosage form requirements: Standards for tablets, capsules, injections, and other pharmaceutical forms.

Relevance to Pharmacovigilance:

Pharmacopoeial information supports pharmacovigilance through:

- Verification of drug composition and potential contaminants
- Understanding pharmaceutical equivalence in generic drug assessments
- Investigating quality-related adverse events
- Evaluating excipient-related reactions
- Assessing reports involving substandard or counterfeit products

6.3 DRUG COMPENDIA AND FORMULARIES

Drug compendia are comprehensive collections of drug information covering multiple therapeutic categories, while **formularies** are curated lists of preferred medications with associated prescribing guidance. These resources bridge basic reference materials and specialized safety resources.

Types and Examples:

National formularies such as the British National Formulary provide clinically focused prescribing guidance updated regularly to reflect current evidence and regulatory changes.

Hospital formularies list medications available within specific healthcare institutions, often with institutional prescribing protocols and restrictions.

Insurance formularies specify medications covered by health insurance plans, organized by tier or preferred status.

Therapeutic compendia like AHFS-DI organize drugs by therapeutic category with comprehensive monographs covering pharmacology, clinical use, and safety.

Content Elements:

Drug compendia typically include:

- Therapeutic indications and off label use
- Dosing recommendations for various patient populations
- Contraindications and precautions
- Adverse reactions organized by frequency and severity
- Drug interactions with clinical significance ratings

- Monitoring parameters and therapeutic guidelines
- Cost information and formulary status

Use in Pharmacovigilance:

Pharmacovigilance professionals consult compendia and formularies to:

- Verify labeled indications versus reported indications
- Assess whether adverse events are documented or unexpected
- Identify drug interactions that may contribute to adverse events
- Understand appropriate dosing to evaluate medication errors
- Compare safety profiles across therapeutic alternatives

6.4 SPECIALIZED RESOURCES FOR ADRs

Specialized adverse drug reaction resources focus specifically on drug safety information, providing comprehensive coverage of adverse effects, toxicology, and risk management. These resources are specifically designed for pharmacovigilance and clinical toxicology applications.

Meyler's Side Effects of Drugs is a comprehensive encyclopedia of adverse drug reactions organized by drug class, providing detailed descriptions of adverse effects with extensive literature references.

Side Effects of Drugs Annual provides yearly updates on newly reported adverse drug reactions and evolving safety information.

Dukes' System Organ Class-based Drug Safety organizes adverse effects by organ system, facilitating differential diagnosis of drug-induced disease.

Stephens' Detection and Evaluation of Adverse Drug Reactions offer methodological guidance on pharmacovigilance principles and signal detection.

Davies' Textbook of Adverse Drug Reactions provides comprehensive clinical descriptions of adverse drug reactions organized by organ system and drug class.

Content Characteristics:

Specialized ADR resources typically provide:

- Detailed descriptions of adverse reaction mechanisms
- Frequency estimates and risk factor identification
- Clinical presentation and diagnostic criteria
- Management and treatment approaches
- Extensive references to primary literature
- Case reports and clinical series

Applications:

These specialized resources support:

- Assessment of causality and biological plausibility
- Identification of risk factors and susceptible populations
- Differential diagnosis of suspected adverse drug reactions
- Literature-based signal validation
- Preparation of safety communications and product labeling

6.5 MICROMEDEX, DRUGDEX

Micromedex is a comprehensive suite of evidence-based clinical databases widely used in healthcare settings for drug information, toxicology, and disease management. The **Drugdex System** within Micromedex provides detailed drug evaluations with particular emphasis on safety, interactions, and comparative effectiveness.

Structure of Drugdex:

Each Drugdex drug evaluation contains standardized sections:

Drug Consults: Concise summaries providing quick answers to common clinical questions about dosing, indications, adverse effects, and interactions.

Dosing and Administration: Detailed dosing recommendations for various indications, patient populations, and clinical scenarios.

Adverse Reaction Evaluations: Comprehensive compilations of reported adverse effects organized by frequency, severity, and organ system, with severity ratings (minor, moderate, severe) and documentation levels (established, probable, suspected).

Drug Interactions: Extensive interaction monographs with severity ratings (contraindicated, major, moderate, minor) and documentation levels (excellent, good, fair, poor).

Pharmacokinetics: Detailed information on absorption, distribution, metabolism, and elimination.

Comparative Efficacy: Evidence-based comparisons of therapeutic alternatives within drug classes.

Off-Label Uses: Evaluation of evidence for non-FDA approved indications with effectiveness ratings.

Evidence-Based Approach:

Drugdex employs a systematic evidence evaluation methodology:

- Comprehensive literature review of primary studies
- Critical appraisal of evidence quality
- Standardized rating scales for efficacy and safety
- Regular updates incorporating new evidence
- Editorial review by clinical experts

Table 11: Drugdex Evidence Rating System

Rating	Meaning
Class I	Evidence from controlled studies
Class IIa	Evidence favors efficacy
Class IIb	Efficacy less well established
Class III	Evidence indicates ineffectiveness

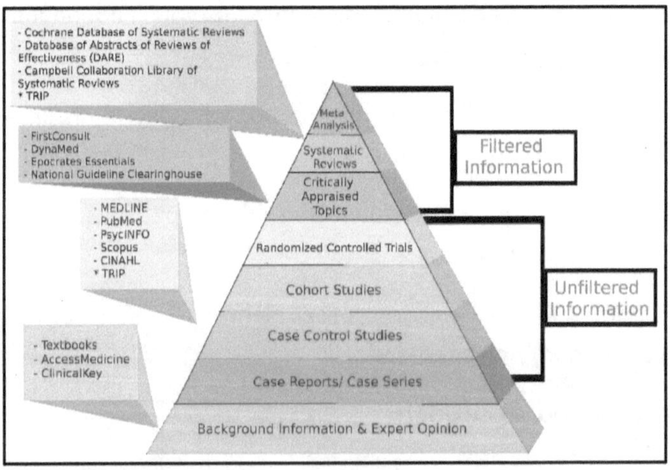

Figure 11: This table presents the Drugdex classification system for evaluating clinical evidence supporting drug uses, providing pharmacovigilance professionals with a framework for assessing the strength of evidence when evaluating labeled and off-label indications.

Pharmacovigilance Applications:

Micromedex and Drugdex support pharmacovigilance through:

- Comprehensive adverse effect profiles for causality assessment

- Interaction evaluations for investigating complex cases
- Toxicology information for overdose and poisoning cases
- Comparative safety data for risk-benefit assessment
- Evidence ratings for evaluating appropriateness of drug use

6.6 WHO PHARMACEUTICALS NEWSLETTER

The **WHO Pharmaceuticals Newsletter** is a bimonthly publication that communicates drug safety information, regulatory decisions, and pharmacovigilance updates from the WHO Programme for International Drug Monitoring and national regulatory authorities worldwide.

Content and Organization:

Each issue contains:

Safety Information: Reports of newly identified adverse drug reactions, safety signals under investigation, and emerging safety concerns from the WHO global database.

Regulatory Decisions: Summaries of regulatory actions taken by national authorities including product withdrawals, label changes, and new contraindications.

International Non-proprietary Names: Lists of proposed and recommended INNs for new substances.

ATC/DDD Updates: Notifications of new ATC classifications and DDD assignments.

Meeting Reports: Summaries of WHO expert committee meetings and pharmacovigilance conferences.

Signal Review: Discussions of signals detected through analysis of VigiBase with expert commentary on clinical significance.

Purpose and Audience:

The Newsletter serves multiple stakeholder groups:

- National pharmacovigilance centers and regulatory authorities
- Healthcare professionals interested in drug safety
- Pharmaceutical industry safety departments
- Academic researchers in pharmacovigilance
- International drug policy organizations

Value in Pharmacovigilance:

The WHO Pharmaceuticals Newsletter provides:

- Early awareness of emerging safety issues globally
- International perspective on regulatory actions
- Access to safety information from diverse healthcare systems
- Standardized nomenclature updates
- Evidence of international recognition of safety signals

6.7 FDA MEDWATCH

FDA MedWatch is the United States Food and Drug Administration's Safety Information and Adverse Event Reporting Program. It serves dual functions: facilitating voluntary reporting of adverse events by healthcare professionals and consumers and communicating important drug safety information to the medical community.

MedWatch Safety Alerts:

The FDA issues several types of safety communications through MedWatch:

Drug Safety Communications: Comprehensive announcements of new safety information requiring public awareness, including new warnings, contraindications, or usage restrictions.

Safety Alerts: Urgent notifications of serious safety issues requiring immediate attention.

Public Health Advisories: Broader safety concerns affecting public health beyond individual products.

Dear Healthcare Provider Letters: Formal communications from manufacturers to healthcare professionals describing safety issues and recommended actions.

Reporting System:

The MedWatch reporting system enables:

- Voluntary reporting by healthcare professionals and consumers
- Confidential submission of adverse event reports
- Online, telephone, mail, and fax reporting options
- Direct data entry into the FDA Adverse Event Reporting System (FAERS)

Pharmacovigilance Applications:

MedWatch supports pharmacovigilance by:

- Providing timely access to FDA safety determinations
- Enabling awareness of regulatory actions affecting product labeling
- Facilitating literature-based signal validation

- Supporting compliance with safety communication requirements
- Informing risk management strategies

6.8 ELECTRONIC DATABASES FOR DRUG SAFETY

Electronic databases provide systematic access to published literature, clinical trial data, and adverse event reports essential for pharmacovigilance literature surveillance, signal validation, and safety assessment.

Bibliographic Databases:

PubMed/MEDLINE: The primary biomedical literature database maintained by the US National Library of Medicine, containing over 35 million citations with coverage from 1946 to present.

Embase: A comprehensive biomedical database with particular strength in drug safety literature, including conference abstracts and European publications.

International Pharmaceutical Abstracts (IPA): Focuses specifically on pharmaceutical literature including pharmacy practice, drug therapy, and pharmacovigilance.

Cochrane Library: Contains systematic reviews and meta-analyses evaluating healthcare interventions including drug safety outcomes.

Safety Databases:

FDA Adverse Event Reporting System (FAERS): Publicly accessible database of adverse event reports submitted to the FDA, enabling signal detection and safety research.

EudraVigilance: European database of suspected adverse drug reaction reports, with public access to aggregate data and signal detection reports.

VigiBase: WHO global database of Individual Case Safety Reports containing over 30 million reports from more than 150 countries.

Clinical Trial Registries:

ClinicalTrials.gov: Registry of clinical studies worldwide, providing access to study protocols, results, and adverse event data from completed trials.

EU Clinical Trials Register: European registry providing information on clinical trials conducted in the European Union.

Search Strategies:

Effective database searching requires:

- Use of controlled vocabulary (MeSH terms, Emtree)
- Boolean operators for combining search concepts
- Field-specific searching (title, abstract, publication type)
- Appropriate filters (date, language, study design)
- Regular update searches to capture new publications

Applications in Literature Surveillance:

Electronic databases support:

- Systematic signal detection through literature monitoring
- Case series identification for signal validation
- Evidence synthesis for safety evaluations
- Competitor product safety monitoring
- Regulatory submission preparation

Understanding the scope, content, and appropriate application of these diverse resources enables pharmacovigilance professionals to conduct comprehensive case evaluations, validate safety signals, and prepare evidence-based safety communications. The integration of traditional reference materials with modern electronic databases reflects the evolution of pharmacovigilance into a data-intensive, evidence-based discipline requiring sophisticated information literacy.

Students must develop proficiency in accessing, evaluating, and synthesizing information from multiple sources to support pharmacovigilance activities in clinical, regulatory, and industrial settings. The resources described in this chapter form the foundation for evidence-based pharmacovigilance practice throughout the product lifecycle.

CHAPTER 7

ESTABLISHING PHARMACOVIGILANCE PROGRAMME

KEY OUTCOMES

Upon completion of this chapter, learners will be able to:

1. Describe the process of establishing pharmacovigilance in a hospital setting
2. Understand the structure and functions of a Hospital Pharmacovigilance Committee
3. Explain the establishment and operation of Drug Safety Department in pharmaceutical industry
4. Describe the Pharmacovigilance System Master File (PSMF) and its regulatory requirements
5. Define the role and responsibilities of the Qualified Person for Pharmacovigilance (QPPV)
6. Understand the role of Contract Research Organizations (CROs) in pharmacovigilance
7. Explain the process of establishing a National Pharmacovigilance Programme
8. Describe Quality Management Systems in pharmacovigilance operations

ABSTRACT

The establishment of effective pharmacovigilance programmes requires systematic planning, organizational structure, resource allocation, and adherence to regulatory requirements. This chapter examines the principles and processes for establishing pharmacovigilance systems in hospital, industrial, and national settings. Hospital pharmacovigilance programmes focus on detecting and managing adverse drug reactions within healthcare institutions through multidisciplinary committees and standardized reporting procedures. Industrial pharmacovigilance departments maintain regulatory compliance, manage global safety databases, and fulfill post-marketing surveillance obligations. The Pharmacovigilance System Master File and Qualified Person for Pharmacovigilance represent key regulatory requirements in the pharmaceutical industry. National pharmacovigilance programmes coordinate drug safety monitoring at the country level, interfacing with international networks and supporting public health decision-making. Quality management systems ensure the reliability, consistency, and regulatory compliance of pharmacovigilance operations across all settings. Understanding these organizational frameworks prepares students for roles in establishing, operating, and improving pharmacovigilance systems throughout their professional careers.

7.1 ESTABLISHING PHARMACOVIGILANCE IN A HOSPITAL

Hospital pharmacovigilance programmes serve as the frontline systems for detecting, documenting, and managing adverse drug reactions in healthcare settings. Establishing an effective hospital-based programme requires administrative support, multidisciplinary collaboration, standardized procedures, and integration with clinical care processes.

Rationale and Objectives:

Hospital pharmacovigilance aims to:

- Detect adverse drug reactions occurring during hospitalization
- Reduce preventable medication-related harm
- Improve prescribing practices through safety feedback
- Generate institutional ADR data for local decision-making
- Contribute to national and international pharmacovigilance systems
- Support medico-legal documentation
- Facilitate medication safety quality improvement

Essential Components:

Leadership and administrative support: Institutional commitment from hospital administration provides necessary resources, authority, and priority for pharmacovigilance activities.

Designated personnel: A pharmacovigilance team including clinical pharmacists, physicians, and nurses coordinates ADR monitoring activities.

Standard Operating Procedures: Written protocols define ADR detection, reporting, assessment, documentation, and follow-up processes.

Reporting mechanisms: Multiple reporting pathways accommodate spontaneous reporting by healthcare professionals and active surveillance by pharmacovigilance personnel.

Documentation systems: Electronic or paper-based systems capture ADR details following standardized formats.

Communication channels: Established pathways disseminate safety information to prescribers, pharmacy, nursing, and administration.

Implementation Steps:

Needs assessment: Evaluate institutional medication use patterns, patient populations, existing medication safety infrastructure, and available resources.

Stakeholder engagement: Involve medical staff, pharmacy department, nursing administration, quality improvement teams, and hospital leadership in programme planning.

Resource allocation: Secure dedicated personnel time, space, equipment, and information technology support.

Training programmes: Educate healthcare professionals on ADR recognition, causality assessment, reporting procedures, and documentation requirements.

Pilot implementation: Begin with focused surveillance in high-risk areas (intensive care units, oncology) to demonstrate feasibility and value.

Expansion and integration: Gradually extend coverage throughout the institution and integrate pharmacovigilance into routine clinical workflows.

Outcome evaluation: Monitor programme performance through metrics such as reporting rates, ADR detection, interventions implemented and prevented harm.

7.2 HOSPITAL PHARMACOVIGILANCE COMMITTEE

The **Hospital Pharmacovigilance Committee** (or Adverse Drug Reaction Monitoring Committee) provides governance, oversight, and multidisciplinary expertise for institutional pharmacovigilance activities. This committee ensures systematic ADR monitoring, guides policy development, and links pharmacovigilance with broader medication safety initiatives.

Composition:

The committee typically includes:

- **Chairperson**: Senior physician or clinical pharmacologist
- **Clinical Pharmacologist**: Expert in drug therapy and ADR assessment
- **Clinical Pharmacists**: Provide pharmaceutical expertise and coordinate surveillance
- **Physician Representatives**: From major clinical departments
- **Nursing Representatives**: Contribute frontline ADR recognition perspectives
- **Quality/Risk Management**: Link pharmacovigilance with patient safety systems
- **Secretary**: Maintains records and coordinates meetings

Functions and Responsibilities:

Policy development: Establish institutional ADR monitoring policies, reporting requirements, and procedural guidelines.

Case review: Evaluate reported ADRs for causality, severity, preventability, and required actions.

Signal identification: Identify patterns or clusters of ADRs suggesting safety concerns.

Intervention recommendations: Propose changes in prescribing practices, formulary decisions, or clinical protocols based on ADR patterns.

Education and awareness: Coordinate training programmes and safety communications for healthcare professionals.

Reporting coordination: Oversee submission of serious ADRs to national pharmacovigilance centres and regulatory authorities.

Performance monitoring: Review programme metrics and recommend improvements.

Meeting Frequency and Documentation:

Committees typically meet monthly or quarterly depending on institutional size and ADR volume. Meeting minutes document cases reviewed, decisions made, interventions recommended, and follow-up actions. Serious or unexpected ADRs may trigger ad hoc meetings for urgent review.

Linkages with Other Committees:

The pharmacovigilance committee coordinates with:

- Pharmacy and Therapeutics Committee for formulary decisions
- Medication Safety Committee for error prevention
- Quality Improvement teams for systems improvement
- Infection Control Committee for antimicrobial safety
- Ethics Committee for research-related ADRs

7.3 ESTABLISHMENT AND OPERATION OF DRUG SAFETY DEPARTMENT IN INDUSTRY

Pharmaceutical and biotechnology companies maintain dedicated **Drug Safety Departments** (also called Pharmacovigilance Departments or Drug Safety Units) responsible for monitoring the safety of their marketed products and investigational compounds. These departments fulfill regulatory obligations, manage safety data, conduct safety assessments, and communicate risks to stakeholders.

Organizational Structure:

Drug Safety Departments vary in size and structure depending on company size, product portfolio, and global footprint. Typical organizational elements include:

Global Safety Leadership: Senior executives (Chief Safety Officer, Vice President of Global Safety) provide strategic direction and regulatory accountability.

Safety Operations: Teams manage case processing, data entry, medical review, and reporting compliance.

Safety Surveillance: Scientists conduct signal detection, aggregate data analysis, and epidemiological studies.

Risk Management: Specialists develop and monitor risk minimization programmes.

Medical Safety: Physicians provide clinical expertise for case assessment and benefit-risk evaluation.

Regulatory Affairs Liaison: Coordinates safety submissions with regulatory authorities.

Information Technology: Supports safety databases and electronic reporting systems.

Quality Assurance: Ensures compliance with regulations and internal standards.

Core Functions:

Case management: Receive, process, and evaluate Individual Case Safety Reports from all sources (clinical trials, spontaneous reports, literature, solicited programmes).

Regulatory reporting: Submit expedited reports of serious adverse events and periodic safety reports to regulatory authorities within mandated timelines.

Safety surveillance: Monitor accumulated safety data to detect signals of new or changing risks.

Safety documentation: Maintain current safety information in product labeling, investigator brochures, and patient materials.

Risk management: Develop, implement, and monitor Risk Evaluation and Mitigation Strategies (REMS) or Risk Management Plans.

Medical information support: Provide safety information responses to healthcare professionals and patients.

Clinical trial safety: Monitor safety in ongoing clinical studies and support data monitoring committees.

Post-authorization safety studies: Conduct observational studies to characterize risks in real-world settings.

Resource Requirements:

Establishing a Drug Safety Department requires:

- Qualified personnel including physicians, pharmacists, nurses, epidemiologists, and data specialists
- Safety database systems compliant with regulatory requirements (E2B standards)
- Document management systems for safety records retention
- Literature surveillance and bibliographic database access
- Standard Operating Procedures covering all processes
- Training programmes for safety personnel
- Quality management systems ensuring compliance

7.4 PHARMACOVIGILANCE SYSTEM MASTER FILE (PSMF)

The **Pharmacovigilance System Master File (PSMF)** is a detailed description of a marketing authorization holder's pharmacovigilance system, required by European regulations for all medicinal products authorized in the European Economic Area. The PSMF provides regulatory authorities with a comprehensive overview of the company's pharmacovigilance capabilities and organizational arrangements.

Regulatory Basis:

The PSMF requirement is established in European Union legislation (Regulation 726/2004 and Directive 2001/83/EC as amended). Marketing authorization holders must maintain a PSMF and make it available to competent authorities upon request. The PSMF must be located in the European Economic Area at the site of the Qualified Person for Pharmacovigilance.

Structure and Content:

The PSMF follows a standardized structure defined in regulatory guidance (GVP Module II):

Part I - Core elements of the pharmacovigilance system applicable to all medicinal products:

- Qualified Person for Pharmacovigilance identification and contact information
- Organizational structure of the pharmacovigilance system
- Sources of safety data and methods for collection
- Computerized systems and databases
- Quality management system elements
- Procedures for signal management

- Periodic safety update report processes
- Risk management system overview
- Mechanisms for collaboration and communication
- Master file location and archiving

Part II - Product-specific elements for each authorized product:

- Marketing authorization details for each product
- Qualified Person for Pharmacovigilance responsible for the product
- Product-specific safety concerns
- Risk management plans
- Summary of ongoing or planned pharmacovigilance activities
- Post-authorization safety study protocols

Maintenance and Updates:

The marketing authorization holder must keep the PSMF up to date, reflecting current organizational structures, procedures, and product-specific information. Changes must be documented promptly, and version control maintained. Regulatory authorities may inspect the PSMF during pharmacovigilance inspections to verify system adequacy and compliance.

7.5 QUALIFIED PERSON FOR PHARMACOVIGILANCE (QPPV)

The **Qualified Person for Pharmacovigilance (QPPV)** is the individual within a marketing authorization holder's organization who has overall responsibility for the pharmacovigilance system and for ensuring appropriate communication with regulatory authorities regarding safety matters. The QPPV role is a regulatory requirement in the European Union and many other jurisdictions.

Qualification Requirements:

The QPPV must:

- Possess appropriate medical or pharmacy qualifications
- Be a resident in the European Economic Area
- Have sufficient knowledge of pharmacovigilance regulations and guidelines
- Have appropriate scientific training and experience
- Be permanently and continuously available to fulfill QPPV responsibilities

Responsibilities:

The QPPV's key responsibilities include:

System oversight: Ensure the marketing authorization holder has an appropriate pharmacovigilance system in place and functioning properly.

PSMF maintenance: Take responsibility for the accuracy and completeness of the Pharmacovigilance System Master File.

Regulatory communication: Serve as the contact point for competent authorities on pharmacovigilance matters.

Compliance assurance: Ensure that obligations for expedited reporting, periodic reporting, and risk management are fulfilled.

Signal management: Oversee the identification, assessment, and communication of safety signals.

Documentation oversight: Ensure appropriate records and documentation are maintained.

Quality system supervision: Oversee quality management systems for pharmacovigilance activities.

Authority and Resources:

The QPPV must have:

- Access to all safety data sources
- Authority to deploy resources for pharmacovigilance activities
- Direct communication with senior management
- Independence to fulfill responsibilities without conflicts of interest
- Support staff and infrastructure adequate for the product portfolio

7.6 CONTRACT RESEARCH ORGANIZATIONS (CROs) IN PHARMACOVIGILANCE

Contract Research Organizations are third-party service providers that perform pharmacovigilance activities on behalf of pharmaceutical companies, biotechnology firms, medical device manufacturers, and other sponsors. CROs enable companies to access specialized expertise, scale resources flexibly, and manage global pharmacovigilance operations efficiently.

Services Provided:

CROs offer a range of pharmacovigilance services:

Case processing: Receipt, data entry, medical review, and regulatory reporting of Individual Case Safety Reports.

Literature surveillance: Systematic monitoring of medical literature for safety information.

Aggregate reporting: Preparation of Periodic Safety Update Reports and Periodic Benefit-Risk Evaluation Reports.

Signal detection: Statistical analysis of safety databases and medical review of potential signals.

Risk management: Development and implementation of Risk Evaluation and Mitigation Strategies and Risk Management Plans.

Post-authorization safety studies: Design, conduct, and analysis of observational safety studies.

Regulatory submissions: Preparation and submission of safety-related regulatory documents.

Safety database management: Maintenance and validation of pharmacovigilance databases.

Training and consulting: Expert guidance on pharmacovigilance regulations, processes, and compliance.

Advantages and Considerations:

Benefits of CRO partnerships:

- Access to specialized pharmacovigilance expertise
- Flexible resource scaling for changing workloads
- Cost efficiencies compared to in-house infrastructure
- Global operational capabilities
- Technology platforms and database systems
- Reduced time-to-market through parallel activities

Important considerations:

- Sponsor retains ultimate responsibility for pharmacovigilance
- Need for robust oversight and quality agreements
- Data security and confidentiality requirements

- Clear definition of roles and responsibilities
- Communication protocols and escalation procedures
- Regular audits to ensure compliance
- Knowledge management and continuity planning

Contractual Arrangements:

Effective CRO partnerships require:

- Detailed contracts specifying services, timelines, and deliverables
- Quality agreements defining standards and compliance expectations
- Standard Operating Procedures for all delegated activities
- Key performance indicators and service level agreements
- Regular performance reviews and governance meetings
- Clear procedures for information exchange and communication

7.7 ESTABLISHING A NATIONAL PROGRAMME

National Pharmacovigilance Programmes coordinate drug safety monitoring at the country level, serving as the interface between healthcare providers, pharmaceutical industry, regulatory authorities, and international pharmacovigilance networks. Establishing an effective national programme requires government commitment, regulatory framework, infrastructure development, and stakeholder engagement.

Prerequisites and Planning:

Successful establishment requires:

Political commitment: Government recognition of pharmacovigilance as a public health priority with allocation of resources.

Regulatory framework: Legal authority for adverse event reporting, data collection, and regulatory action based on safety findings.

Institutional home: Designation of a host institution (regulatory authority, ministry of health, academic center) with appropriate governance.

Resource mobilization: Securing funding for personnel, information technology, training, and operations.

Stakeholder mapping: Identifying healthcare providers, hospitals, pharmaceutical companies, patient organizations, and other partners.

Capacity assessment: Evaluating existing infrastructure, trained personnel, and information systems.

Implementation Strategy:

Phase 1 - Foundation Building:

- Establish national pharmacovigilance center with core staff
- Develop legal and regulatory framework
- Create Standard Operating Procedures
- Implement adverse event reporting system
- Establish database for case collection

Phase 2 - Network Development:

- Identify and train regional pharmacovigilance centers
- Establish sentinel sites in major hospitals

- Engage healthcare professional associations
- Develop reporting mechanisms (paper, online, mobile)
- Create communication channels for safety information dissemination

Phase 3 - System Strengthening:

- Expand surveillance coverage nationally
- Enhance signal detection capabilities
- Develop risk communication strategies
- Integrate with regulatory decision-making
- Link with international pharmacovigilance systems

Phase 4 - Maturation and Innovation:

- Implement active surveillance systems
- Conduct pharmacoepidemiological studies
- Develop risk management capabilities
- Enhance stakeholder engagement
- Contribute to international signal detection

International Collaboration:

National programmes benefit from participation in:

WHO Programme for International Drug Monitoring: Membership provides access to VigiBase global database, signal detection tools, training resources, and international expertise.

Regional networks: Collaboration with neighboring countries enables resource sharing and comparative safety analysis.

Technical partnerships: Relationships with established programmes provide mentoring, training opportunities, and technical assistance.

7.8 STRUCTURE AND FUNCTION OF NATIONAL PHARMACOVIGILANCE PROGRAMME

An effective national pharmacovigilance programme requires appropriate organizational structure, clear functional responsibilities, and integration with the broader healthcare and regulatory ecosystem.

Organizational Structure:

National Pharmacovigilance Centre: Central coordinating body responsible for overall programme management, typically situated within the national medicines' regulatory authority or as an independent agency.

Key components include:

Leadership and governance: Director and advisory committee providing strategic direction

Technical units: Teams for case management, signal detection, risk assessment, and communication

Quality assurance: Unit ensuring compliance and data quality

Training and capacity building: Team developing educational programmes

Information technology: Technical support for databases and reporting systems

Regional/Peripheral Centers: Pharmacovigilance focal points in different geographic areas or major hospitals serving as data collection sites and local training hubs.

Sentinel Sites: Selected healthcare facilities with enhanced surveillance capabilities providing high-quality ADR reports.

Core Functions:

Data collection and management: Receive, process, and manage adverse event reports from healthcare professionals, consumers, and pharmaceutical companies.

Causality assessment: Evaluate reported cases to determine likelihood of causal relationship between drug and adverse event.

Signal detection and evaluation: Systematically analyze accumulated data to identify potential safety signals and assess their public health significance.

Risk assessment: Evaluate benefit-risk balance of medicinal products based on evolving safety information.

Regulatory action: Recommend or implement regulatory measures (label changes, restrictions, withdrawals) based on safety assessments.

Communication: Disseminate drug safety information to healthcare professionals, patients, and the public through safety alerts, newsletters, and educational materials.

International reporting: Share serious and unexpected adverse event reports with WHO and other international partners.

Research and training: Conduct pharmacoepidemiological research and provide training to healthcare professionals and stakeholders.

Performance Indicators:

Programme effectiveness is monitored through:

- Number of ADR reports received (absolute and per million population)
- Report quality and completeness
- Timeliness of report processing and regulatory reporting
- Number of signals detected and evaluated

- Regulatory actions taken based on safety findings
- Coverage of healthcare facilities participating in reporting
- Healthcare professional awareness and engagement
- Contribution to international pharmacovigilance

Integration with Healthcare System:

Effective programmes integrate with:

- Medical education curricula for healthcare professionals
- Hospital medication safety systems
- Clinical practice guideline development
- Health technology assessment processes
- Essential medicines selection
- Pharmaceutical procurement and supply systems

7.9 QUALITY MANAGEMENT SYSTEMS IN PHARMACOVIGILANCE

Quality Management Systems (QMS) in pharmacovigilance ensure that all activities are conducted reliably, consistently, and in compliance with regulatory requirements. A robust QMS encompasses documented procedures, performance monitoring, continuous improvement, and accountability mechanisms.

Principles of Pharmaceutical Quality:

Pharmacovigilance quality systems are based on:

Regulatory compliance: Adherence to applicable laws, regulations, and guidelines (ICH, GVP, FDA regulations).

Scientific rigor: Application of sound scientific principles in data collection, assessment, and interpretation.

Consistency: Standardized processes ensuring uniform handling of similar situations.

Transparency: Clear documentation enabling traceability and auditability.

Continuous improvement: Systematic identification and correction of deficiencies.

Risk-based approach: Prioritization of quality efforts based on potential impact on patient safety and regulatory compliance.

Key Elements:

Standard Operating Procedures (SOPs): Written instructions describing detailed procedures for all pharmacovigilance activities including case processing, medical review, reporting, signal detection, and documentation.

Training programmes: Systematic initial and ongoing training ensuring personnel have appropriate knowledge and competencies for their roles.

Document management: Systems for creation, review, approval, distribution, and archiving of pharmacovigilance documents.

Data quality assurance: Processes ensuring accuracy, completeness, and consistency of safety data through validation, quality checks, and reconciliation.

Performance monitoring: Key performance indicators tracking timeliness, accuracy, and completeness of pharmacovigilance activities.

Audit programmes: Regular internal audits and inspections evaluating compliance with procedures and identifying improvement opportunities.

Corrective and Preventive Actions (CAPA): Systematic investigation of deviations, implementation of corrections, and prevention of recurrence.

Change control: Formal processes for evaluating, approving, and implementing changes to systems, procedures, or processes.

Quality Metrics:

Common pharmacovigilance quality indicators include:

Timeliness metrics:

- Percentage of expedited reports submitted within regulatory timelines
- Time from receipt to database entry
- Time from receipt to medical review completion

Quality metrics:

- Percentage of reports meeting data quality standards
- Accuracy of coding (adverse events, drugs, outcomes)
- Completeness of case documentation

Compliance metrics:

- Adherence to SOPs
- Training completion rates
- Audit findings and CAPA closure rates

Regulatory Inspections:

Regulatory authorities conduct pharmacovigilance inspections to verify:

- Adequacy of pharmacovigilance systems
- Compliance with regulatory requirements
- Data integrity and quality
- Effectiveness of quality management systems

- Proper functioning of oversight mechanisms

Inspection readiness requires:

- Complete and current documentation
- Availability of records and audit trails
- Trained personnel familiar with systems and procedures
- Demonstration of continuous monitoring and improvement

Table 12: Key Quality Management Components in Pharmacovigilance

Component	Purpose	Key Activities
SOPs	Standardize procedures	Document processes, maintain versions, ensure accessibility
Training	Ensure competency	Initial training, ongoing education, competency assessment
Quality Control	Verify data quality	Data validation, quality checks, error correction
Audits	Assess compliance	Internal audits, vendor audits, inspection preparation
CAPA	Drive improvement	Investigate deviations, implement corrections, prevent recurrence
Metrics	Monitor performance	Track KPIs, analyze trends, report to management

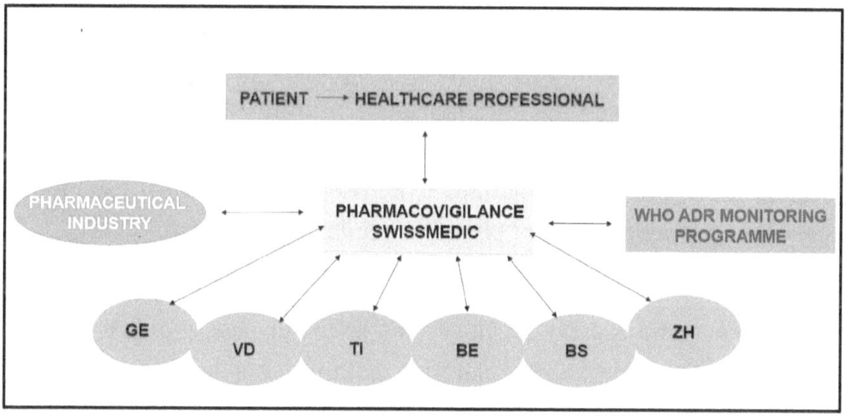

Figure. 12: This table summarizes the essential components of a pharmacovigilance quality management system, illustrating how multiple quality elements work together to ensure reliable, compliant, and continuously improving drug safety operations.

Quality Culture:

Beyond formal systems, effective pharmacovigilance requires a quality culture characterized by:

- Management commitment to quality and patient safety
- Personnel accountability for quality in daily work
- Open communication about errors and improvement opportunities
- Recognition that quality is everyone's responsibility
- Continuous learning and adaptation based on experience

Hospital pharmacovigilance programmes bring drug safety monitoring directly into clinical care settings, enabling real-time detection of adverse reactions and immediate intervention to prevent harm. The Hospital Pharmacovigilance Committee provides multidisciplinary governance and links safety monitoring with institutional quality improvement.

Industrial pharmacovigilance departments fulfill complex regulatory obligations throughout the product lifecycle, from clinical development through post-marketing surveillance. The Pharmacovigilance System Master File and Qualified Person for Pharmacovigilance represent key regulatory accountability mechanisms ensuring that pharmaceutical companies maintain robust safety monitoring systems. Contract Research Organizations provide specialized expertise and operational capabilities that enable flexible, efficient pharmacovigilance operations.

National pharmacovigilance programmes coordinate drug safety monitoring at the country level, serving as the critical interface between healthcare providers, regulatory authorities, and international pharmacovigilance networks. Establishing effective national programmes requires sustained political commitment, appropriate regulatory frameworks, infrastructure development, and integration with broader healthcare systems.

Quality management systems provide the foundation for reliable, compliant pharmacovigilance operations across all settings. Through documented procedures, systematic training, performance monitoring, and continuous improvement, quality systems ensure that pharmacovigilance activities consistently meet regulatory requirements and scientific standards.

CHAPTER 8

VACCINE SAFETY SURVEILLANCE

KEY OUTCOMES

Upon completion of this chapter, learners will be able to:

1. Understand the fundamental principles of vaccine pharmacovigilance and how they differ from drug safety monitoring.
2. Explain the unique aspects of vaccine safety monitoring, including population-level surveillance and AEFI investigations.
3. Describe the importance of vaccine safety monitoring in maintaining public trust and sustaining immunization coverage.
4. Evaluate the benefit-risk assessment process used to determine vaccine safety profiles.
5. Recognize the role of global initiatives such as WHO's Global Vaccine Safety Initiative (GVSI) and GACVS in harmonizing safety monitoring worldwide.
6. Appreciate how transparent communication and data-driven safety systems contribute to public confidence in vaccines

ABSTRACT

Vaccine safety surveillance is a cornerstone of modern immunization programmes, ensuring that vaccines administered to millions worldwide remain safe, effective, and trusted. As vaccines are preventive biological products given to healthy individuals, their safety standards must be exceptionally high. This chapter explores the scientific and operational aspects of vaccine pharmacovigilance, detailing post-licensure safety monitoring systems, global reporting networks, and mechanisms for detecting adverse events following immunization (AEFI). It discusses the importance of maintaining public confidence through transparent communication, continuous benefit-risk evaluation, and collaboration among regulatory authorities, healthcare professionals, and international agencies such as the World Health Organization (WHO). Furthermore, the chapter examines global initiatives that strengthen vaccine safety monitoring, especially in the context of rapid vaccine development, emergency use authorizations, and emerging infectious diseases.

8.1 Vaccine Pharmacovigilance

Unique Aspects of Vaccine Safety Monitoring

Vaccine pharmacovigilance refers to the science and activities related to detecting, assessing, understanding, and preventing adverse effects or any other vaccine-related problems. Unlike conventional pharmaceuticals, vaccines are administered to large populations, often healthy individuals, including children, pregnant women, and the elderly. Consequently, the tolerance for safety issues is far lower, and the expectations for transparency and accountability are significantly higher.

The unique aspects of vaccine safety monitoring include:

1. **Population-wide Administration:**

Vaccines are given to healthy populations, sometimes in mass immunization campaigns. Hence, even rare adverse reactions can become visible when millions of doses are administered.

2. **Programmatic Factors:**

Adverse events can result not only from the vaccine itself but also from errors in handling, storage, or administration. Such programmatic errors (e.g., cold chain failure, contamination, or incorrect injection technique) must be differentiated from true vaccine reactions.

3. **Temporal Association vs. Causality:**

Because vaccinations are scheduled events, temporal associations between vaccination and illness are common. Distinguishing coincidental events from causally related adverse reactions requires robust data collection and scientific analysis.

4. **Public Sensitivity:**

Public perception plays a crucial role in vaccine acceptance. A single reported adverse event, even if coincidental, can influence community trust. Hence, effective communication and prompt investigation are essential.

5. **Post-Licensure Surveillance:**

Pre-licensure clinical trials may not detect rare adverse events due to limited sample sizes. Post-marketing surveillance is therefore critical to detect and investigate signals that arise once a vaccine is in widespread use.

Importance in Immunization Programmes

The effectiveness of national immunization programmes relies not only on vaccine efficacy but also on the sustained confidence of the population in vaccine safety. Vaccine pharmacovigilance ensures that safety issues are rapidly detected and addressed, maintaining the credibility of health authorities and preventing disruptions to immunization schedules.

Through systematic monitoring and investigation of AEFIs, health authorities can:

- Identify and correct programmatic errors, improving service quality.
- Detect new or unexpected adverse events early.
- Assess risk factors associated with specific vaccines or populations.
- Support evidence-based decision-making for vaccine policy updates.

National regulatory agencies, such as the Central Drugs Standard Control Organization (CDSCO) in India, and global partners like the WHO and UNICEF, work collaboratively to enhance pharmacovigilance systems. Their combined efforts help ensure that vaccines remain safe and effective, and that immunization programmes continue to protect populations worldwide.

8.2 IMPORTANCE OF VACCINE SAFETY MONITORING

Vaccine safety monitoring serves as the cornerstone of public trust in immunization programs. Despite extensive pre-licensure testing, clinical trials cannot detect very rare adverse events occurring in fewer than 1 in 10,000 recipients. Post-marketing surveillance becomes essential for identifying these uncommon but potentially serious reactions when vaccines reach millions of individuals.

Public Health Impact

The success of vaccination programs depends critically on maintaining high coverage rates. Even minor safety concerns, whether substantiated or not, can dramatically reduce vaccine acceptance and lead to disease resurgence. Historical examples demonstrate how safety controversies have resulted in decreased immunization rates and subsequent outbreaks of preventable diseases. Robust safety monitoring systems provide evidence-based reassurance to healthcare providers and the public, supporting informed decision-making.

Scientific Rationale

Pre-licensure trials typically involve 10,000 to 30,000 participants and cannot detect adverse events with incidence rates below 1 in 10,000. Post-marketing surveillance monitoring millions of vaccinations can identify rare events and evaluate safety in diverse populations including pregnant women, elderly individuals, and immunocompromised persons often excluded from clinical trials.

Continuous monitoring allows detection of safety signals related to specific vaccine lots, manufacturing changes, or interactions with newly introduced vaccines. Long-term safety assessment extends beyond immediate post-vaccination periods to evaluate delayed adverse events and cumulative effects of multiple immunizations.

Programmatic Benefits

Effective vaccine safety monitoring strengthens immunization programs by identifying and correcting immunization errors, improving vaccine storage and handling practices, and enhancing training for healthcare providers. The data generated inform policy decisions regarding vaccine schedules, contraindications, and target populations.

Safety surveillance contributes to vaccine development by providing real-world evidence of safety profiles, supporting label updates, and guiding formulation improvements. This continuous feedback loop between surveillance and product development enhances overall vaccine quality and safety.

8.3 VACCINATION FAILURE - TYPES AND CAUSES

Vaccination failure occurs when an immunized individual fails to develop adequate protection against the target disease or develops the disease despite previous immunization. Understanding vaccination failure is essential for distinguishing true vaccine-related adverse events from inadequate immunological response or programmatic issues.

Types of Vaccination Failure

Primary Vaccine Failure occurs when the vaccine fails to induce an adequate immune response after the initial vaccination series. This represents a failure in the immunization process itself, where the recipient does not develop protective antibody levels or cellular immunity despite proper vaccine administration. Primary failure rates vary by vaccine type, ranging from 2-10% for most routine vaccines. Factors contributing to primary failure include individual immunological characteristics, genetic variations in immune response, immunodeficiency conditions, and improper vaccine storage or handling.

Secondary Vaccine Failure develops when initial immunization produces adequate immunity that subsequently wanes over time, leaving the individual susceptible to infection. This represents successful initial immunization followed by declining protection. Secondary failure manifests as breakthrough infections occurring months or years after vaccination when antibody levels fall below protective thresholds. The rate of immunity decline varies by vaccine, with some providing lifelong protection while others require booster doses.

Causes of Vaccination Failure

Vaccination failures arise from multiple factors categorized into vaccine-related, host-related, and program-related causes. Understanding these factors enables targeted interventions to improve immunization effectiveness.

Vaccine-Related Factors include manufacturing defects affecting potency, improper formulation, or contamination. Storage and handling errors represent major causes, particularly cold chain failures where vaccines are exposed to temperatures outside the recommended range. Expired vaccines lose potency and fail to induce adequate immunity.

Some vaccine types are inherently less immunogenic, requiring multiple doses or adjuvants to achieve protection.

Host-Related Factors significantly influence vaccine response. Age affects immunological competence, with very young infants and elderly individuals showing reduced responses. Immunodeficiency conditions, whether congenital or acquired, impair vaccine-induced immunity. Concurrent infections or chronic diseases may interfere with immune response. Genetic factors determine individual variation in vaccine immunogenicity. Malnutrition compromises immune function and vaccine effectiveness.

Program-Related Factors encompass administration errors including incorrect dose, wrong route of administration, or improper injection technique. Inadequate number of doses in multi-dose schedules results in incomplete immunity. Inappropriate timing between doses affects immune response development. Simultaneous administration of certain vaccines or immunoglobulins may interfere with immunogenicity

Clinical Manifestations

Vaccination failure manifests as susceptibility to the target disease despite immunization history. Breakthrough infections may present with typical disease symptoms or modified presentations. Laboratory confirmation often reveals absence of protective antibody levels. Documentation of complete vaccination history distinguishes true vaccine failure from incomplete immunization.

8.4 ADVERSE EVENTS FOLLOWING IMMUNIZATION (AEFI)

Adverse Events Following Immunization (AEFI) represent any untoward medical occurrence that follows immunization and does not necessarily have a causal relationship with the vaccine. This broad definition ensures comprehensive surveillance capturing all health events temporally associated with vaccination, enabling thorough investigation to determine actual causality.

Definition and Scope

AEFI encompasses any unfavorable or unintended sign, abnormal laboratory finding, symptom, or disease temporally associated with vaccination, whether or not considered causally related to the vaccine. This inclusive definition differs from adverse drug reactions, which imply causality. The temporal window for AEFI reporting typically extends from the time of vaccination to 30 days post-immunization, though specific events may be monitored for longer periods.

The scope includes local reactions at injection sites, systemic reactions affecting the body generally, allergic or hypersensitivity reactions, and serious events requiring hospitalization. AEFI surveillance also captures program errors, anxiety-related reactions, and coincidental events occurring by chance after vaccination.

Common AEFI Types

Local Reactions occur at the injection site and represent the most frequent AEFI category. Pain, redness, and swelling typically appear within hours of vaccination and resolve within days. Induration or hardening at the injection site may persist longer. Extensive limb swelling occasionally occurs, particularly with booster doses. Local reactions generally indicate appropriate immune response rather than safety concerns.

Systemic Reactions affect the body generally and include fever, irritability, drowsiness, loss of appetite, headache, myalgia, and fatigue. These reactions typically begin within 24-48 hours of vaccination and resolve spontaneously within days. Fever represents a common systemic reaction, particularly in young children, reflecting immune system activation.

Allergic Reactions range from mild urticaria to severe anaphylaxis. Immediate hypersensitivity reactions occurring within minutes to hours of vaccination require emergency intervention. Delayed-type hypersensitivity reactions may appear days after immunization. True anaphylaxis, though rare (approximately 1 per million doses), represents a serious AEFI requiring immediate treatment.

Serious AEFI include events causing hospitalization, significant disability, life-threatening conditions, or death. Examples include intussusception following rotavirus vaccine, Guillain-Barré syndrome, encephalopathy, or severe allergic reactions. Serious AEFI require mandatory reporting and thorough investigation regardless of suspected causality.

Table 13: Classification of AEFI by Severity

Severity Level	Description	Examples
Mild	Minor discomfort, no interference with daily activities	Local pain, mild fever <38.5°C, irritability
Moderate	Discomfort interfering with daily activities, may require medical attention	High fever >39°C, extensive local swelling, persistent crying >3 hours
Severe	Medically significant, requires hospitalization or causes significant disability	Anaphylaxis, seizures, encephalopathy, death

8.5 AEFI CLASSIFICATION

AEFI classification systems organize adverse events into categories based on causality, enabling systematic analysis and appropriate response. The WHO classification system, widely adopted globally, provides a standardized framework for categorizing AEFI according to underlying causes.

WHO AEFI Classification System

The classification distinguishes five major categories based on causal relationships between vaccination and adverse events.

Vaccine Product-Related Reaction occurs due to inherent properties of the vaccine product when properly manufactured and administered. These reactions result from the vaccine's biological or pharmacological characteristics. Examples include local inflammation from adjuvants, fever following measles-containing vaccines, or lymphadenopathy after BCG vaccination. These reactions are typically predictable, documented in product information, and accepted as part of the vaccine's safety profile.

Vaccine Quality Defect-Related Reaction results from manufacturing or handling defects compromising vaccine quality. Contamination during production, incorrect formulation, or degradation from improper storage causes these reactions. Quality defect-related reactions may affect entire vaccine lots and require immediate product recall and investigation. Examples include abscess formation from contaminated vaccines or inadequate immune response from potency loss.

Immunization Error-Related Reaction arises from inappropriate vaccine administration, handling, or storage constituting deviations from recommended procedures. Administration errors include wrong dose, incorrect route, expired vaccine use, or improper injection technique. Storage errors involve cold chain failures. These preventable reactions reflect programmatic weaknesses requiring corrective interventions.

Immunization Anxiety-Related Reaction results from psychological responses to the immunization process rather than vaccine properties. Anxiety-related reactions include vasovagal syncope, hyperventilation, or psychogenic symptoms. These reactions may occur before, during, or after vaccination and can spread through groups (mass psychogenic illness). Recognition prevents misattribution to vaccine properties.

Coincidental Event occurs by temporal association with vaccination but lacks causal relationship. These events would have occurred regardless of immunization. Distinguishing coincidental events from true vaccine reactions requires careful investigation considering background disease rates and temporal patterns.

Practical Application of Classification

Classification determines appropriate response strategies. Vaccine product-related reactions may warrant label updates or formulation modifications. Quality defect-related reactions trigger product recalls and manufacturing investigations. Immunization error-related reactions require training interventions and procedural improvements. Anxiety-related reactions benefit from improved preparation and counseling. Coincidental events require public communication explaining lack of causality.

Table 14: AEFI Classification Decision Tree

Investigation Finding	Classification Category
Reaction consistent with vaccine properties, proper administration	Vaccine product-related
Multiple cases from same vaccine lot, manufacturing issue identified	Vaccine quality defect-related
Deviation from immunization protocols identified	Immunization error-related
Psychogenic mechanism, no organic cause	Immunization anxiety-related
Event expected in population regardless of vaccination	Coincidental event

8.6 AEFI REPORTING AND INVESTIGATION

Systematic AEFI reporting and investigation form the operational foundation of vaccine safety surveillance. Robust reporting systems detect safety signals while thorough investigations determine causality and guide appropriate responses.

AEFI Reporting Systems

Effective reporting systems incorporate multiple components ensuring comprehensive surveillance. Healthcare providers represent primary reporters, with mandatory reporting requirements for serious AEFI. Vaccine manufacturers maintain pharmacovigilance systems reporting suspected adverse events to regulatory authorities. Parents and vaccine recipients contribute through patient-reported outcome systems. Regulatory authorities receive reports from all sources, maintaining national databases.

Reporting mechanisms include standardized forms capturing essential information: patient demographics, vaccination details (vaccine name, manufacturer, lot number, dose, route), event description (symptoms, onset time, severity, outcome), relevant medical history, and concomitant medications. Electronic reporting systems facilitate rapid data transmission and analysis.

Investigation Process

AEFI investigation follows systematic protocols ensuring thorough evaluation while maintaining standardization across cases. The process begins with immediate notification for serious events, particularly deaths, life-threatening reactions, or cluster events affecting multiple recipients.

Initial Assessment involves collecting comprehensive information about the event, reviewing medical records, and interviewing healthcare providers and family members. Investigators verify vaccination details, confirm event occurrence, and document temporal relationships.

Clinical Evaluation includes physical examination when applicable, review of laboratory and diagnostic test results, and assessment of alternative explanations. Medical experts evaluate whether the clinical presentation matches known vaccine-related reactions or suggests other causes.

Causality Assessment determines the likelihood of causal relationship between vaccination and the adverse event. The WHO causality assessment algorithm considers multiple factors including temporal relationship, biological plausibility, previous evidence of vaccine-event association, alternative explanations, and rechallenge information when available.

Causality categories include:

Consistent with causal association when strong evidence supports vaccine causation, temporal relationship is appropriate, biological plausibility exists, and alternative explanations are excluded.

Indeterminate when insufficient evidence exists to support or refute causation, investigation reveals conflicting findings, or critical information is unavailable.

Inconsistent with causal association when evidence strongly suggests alternative causes, temporal relationship is incompatible, or biological implausibility exists.

Field Investigation

Serious events or clusters trigger field investigations examining vaccination practices, vaccine storage and handling, and program implementation quality. Investigators observe immunization sessions, review cold chain records, and interview healthcare staff. Vaccine samples may be retrieved for laboratory testing.

Response and Follow-up

Investigation findings determine appropriate responses. Confirmed vaccine quality defects necessitate product recalls and manufacturing investigations. Identified immunization errors prompt immediate corrective actions, staff retraining, and procedural modifications. Confirmed vaccine product-related reactions may warrant label updates, communication to healthcare providers, or policy changes. Results are communicated to reporters, added to surveillance databases, and shared with relevant stakeholders.

8.7 WHO GLOBAL ADVISORY COMMITTEE ON VACCINE SAFETY

The WHO Global Advisory Committee on Vaccine Safety (GACVS) serves as the premier international body providing independent, authoritative guidance on vaccine safety issues with global implications. Established by WHO in 1999, GACVS reviews vaccine safety concerns, evaluates scientific evidence, and advises WHO on policy matters affecting vaccine safety worldwide.

Structure and Composition

GACVS comprises 14 international experts selected for their specialized knowledge in fields including vaccinology, pediatrics, internal medicine, pharmacovigilance, epidemiology, public health, immunology, and drug regulation. Members serve four-year terms and participate in their individual capacity rather than representing organizations or countries. This independence ensures objective, science-based assessments free from conflicts of interest.

Functions and Responsibilities

GACVS conducts regular reviews of vaccines in widespread use, evaluating safety data from multiple sources including national surveillance systems, clinical studies, and spontaneous reporting systems. The committee responds to urgent safety signals requiring rapid assessment and guidance. Reviews address specific vaccines, particular adverse events, or safety issues affecting vaccine programs globally.

The committee evaluates causality for serious adverse events, considering biological plausibility, epidemiological evidence, clinical data, and laboratory findings. GACVS develops recommendations for WHO and member states regarding vaccine safety monitoring, risk minimization strategies, and communication approaches.

Assessment Process

GACVS meetings occur biannually, though emergency sessions address urgent issues. The committee receives comprehensive evidence reviews prepared by WHO staff, including systematic literature reviews, surveillance data summaries, and country reports. External experts present specialized information. Committee members critically evaluate evidence quality, identify knowledge gaps, and reach consensus conclusions.

Global Impact

GACVS conclusions influence vaccine policies worldwide. When safety concerns emerge, GACVS assessments provide evidence-based guidance helping countries make informed decisions. The committee's endorsement of vaccine safety reassures public health officials and maintains confidence in immunization programs. Conversely, identification of legitimate safety concerns prompts appropriate precautionary measures.

Recent Contributions

GACVS has addressed safety issues including narcolepsy following H1N1 vaccines, yellow fever vaccine-associated viscerotropic disease, rotavirus vaccine and intussusception, and HPV vaccine safety profiles. During the COVID-19 pandemic, GACVS provided ongoing safety assessments of novel vaccines, addressing rare adverse events like thrombosis with thrombocytopenia syndrome and myocarditis.

Table 15: GACVS Safety Signal Evaluation Framework

Evaluation Component	Assessment Criteria
Temporal Association	Time relationship between vaccination and event onset
Biological Plausibility	Scientific mechanism explaining causation
Epidemiological Evidence	Population-based studies showing statistical association
Individual Case Evaluation	Clinical features, alternative diagnoses, rechallenge data
Consistency	Similar findings across different populations and studies

8.8 NATIONAL AEFI SURVEILLANCE PROGRAMME IN INDIA

India's National AEFI Surveillance Programme represents a comprehensive system for monitoring vaccine safety within one of the world's largest immunization programs. Integrated with the Universal Immunization Programme (UIP), the AEFI surveillance system protects public health while maintaining confidence in vaccination.

Program Structure

The National AEFI Surveillance system operates through a hierarchical structure extending from national to district levels. The National AEFI Committee, comprising experts in pediatrics, immunization, epidemiology, and pharmacovigilance, oversees the program and reviews serious AEFI. State AEFI committees conduct regional oversight and investigate serious events within their jurisdictions. District AEFI committees perform initial investigations and manage routine surveillance.

Reporting Mechanisms

India employs multi-tiered reporting capturing AEFI at various healthcare levels. Healthcare workers at immunization sites report all serious AEFI immediately through designated channels. Minor AEFI are documented and reported through routine mechanisms. The program emphasizes zero reporting, where facilities report absence of AEFI, confirming active surveillance.

Classification of AEFI for Reporting

The program prioritizes reporting based on severity. **Minor AEFI** include local reactions and mild systemic reactions not requiring medical intervention. **Serious AEFI** encompass any event causing hospitalization, medically significant disability, threat to life, or death. Serious AEFI require immediate notification within 24 hours.

Investigation Protocol

Serious AEFI trigger structured investigations following standardized protocols. District rapid response teams conduct initial investigations within 48 hours, collecting clinical information, reviewing vaccination records, and assessing program implementation. State committees review investigation findings and classify events using WHO causality assessment.

National committee reviews include deaths, cluster events, or cases with significant public health implications. Expert panels evaluate medical evidence, determine causality, and recommend actions.

Causality Assessment

India follows WHO causality assessment methodology, classifying events as consistent causal association, indeterminate, inconsistent causal association, or unclassifiable. This standardized approach enables comparison with global data and ensures consistent decision-making.

Quality Assurance

The program implements quality assurance measures including regular training for healthcare workers, supervision of immunization sessions, cold chain monitoring, and vaccine quality testing. Adverse event monitoring integrates with broader program quality assessment.

Communication Strategy

The National AEFI program emphasizes transparent communication. Investigation findings are shared with healthcare providers, media, and the public. Regular bulletins summarize surveillance data. Crisis communication protocols address public concerns during safety events.

Program Impact

Since implementation, the National AEFI Surveillance Programme has strengthened vaccine safety monitoring across India. The system detects safety signals, identifies programmatic weaknesses, and maintains public trust. Integration with the Pharmacovigilance Programme of India (PvPI) enhances overall pharmacovigilance capacity.

8.9 BRIGHTON COLLABORATION CASE DEFINITIONS

The Brighton Collaboration represents a global voluntary network developing standardized case definitions for adverse events following immunization. Established in 2000, Brighton Collaboration addresses the critical need for uniform terminology and diagnostic criteria enabling meaningful comparison of vaccine safety data across studies, surveillance systems, and countries.

Purpose and Rationale

Prior to Brighton Collaboration, inconsistent AEFI definitions prevented accurate comparison of safety data from different sources.

Variations in diagnostic criteria, terminology, and severity grading complicated meta-analyses and global safety assessments. Standardized case definitions enable researchers and surveillance systems worldwide to identify and classify AEFI consistently.

Case Definition Development

Brighton Collaboration employs rigorous methodology for developing case definitions. Working groups comprising international experts review existing literature, clinical criteria, and diagnostic standards for specific adverse events. Draft definitions undergo extensive peer review and field testing. Final definitions balance scientific rigor with practical applicability across diverse healthcare settings.

Definition Structure

Each Brighton case definition follows a standardized format including clear event description, diagnostic criteria organized by certainty level, and guidance for data collection. Definitions specify major and minor criteria for diagnosis. Events are classified into levels of diagnostic certainty based on available evidence:

Level 1 (highest certainty) requires comprehensive diagnostic criteria with confirmatory testing. **Level 2** represents high probability with most but not all confirmatory evidence. **Level 3** indicates moderate evidence supporting the diagnosis. **Level 4** (lowest certainty) includes reported events with minimal diagnostic confirmation. This tiered approach accommodates varying resource availability while maintaining diagnostic rigor.

Priority AEFI Definitions

Brighton Collaboration has developed definitions for numerous AEFI including anaphylaxis, Guillain-Barré syndrome, intussusception, encephalitis/encephalopathy, seizures, thrombocytopenia, myocarditis / pericarditis, narcolepsy, and acute disseminated encephalomyelitis.

Additional definitions address local reactions, fever, and other common events.

Application in Surveillance

National surveillance systems incorporate Brighton definitions to standardize AEFI identification and classification. Clinical trials use definitions for consistent adverse event reporting across study sites. Meta-analyses apply definitions to ensure included studies employ comparable diagnostic criteria.

Global Impact

Brighton Collaboration case definitions have become the international standard for vaccine safety surveillance. Regulatory authorities reference Brighton definitions in safety assessments. WHO recommends Brighton definitions for global vaccine safety monitoring. The standardization has substantially improved quality and comparability of vaccine safety data worldwide.

Limitations and Challenges

Implementation challenges include requirement for specialized diagnostic testing not universally available, complexity of some definitions limiting applicability in resource-limited settings, and need for trained personnel to apply definitions correctly. Ongoing revisions address these limitations while maintaining scientific rigor.

Future Directions

Brighton Collaboration continues expanding its portfolio of case definitions, addressing emerging vaccines and newly recognized adverse events. The initiative promotes capacity building for proper definition implementation. Integration with electronic health records and automated surveillance systems enhances definition utility.

Vaccine safety surveillance represents an essential pillar of public health protection, ensuring that immunization programs achieve maximum disease prevention while minimizing risks. This chapter has comprehensively examined the specialized field of vaccine pharmacovigilance, highlighting unique challenges inherent in monitoring products administered to predominantly healthy populations. The distinction between vaccination failure and genuine adverse events underscores the complexity of vaccine safety assessment, requiring sophisticated surveillance systems and rigorous investigation protocols.

Adverse Events Following Immunization encompass diverse manifestations ranging from minor local reactions to serious systemic events. The WHO classification system provides a rational framework for categorizing AEFI based on underlying causes, enabling appropriate responses whether addressing product defects, programmatic errors, or coincidental events. Systematic reporting and investigation protocols ensure thorough evaluation of each event, with causality assessment determining true vaccine-related reactions.

International collaboration through mechanisms like the WHO Global Advisory Committee on Vaccine Safety strengthens global vaccine safety monitoring, providing evidence-based guidance during safety controversies. National programs, exemplified by India's AEFI surveillance system, demonstrate how systematic monitoring operates within large-scale immunization initiatives. The Brighton Collaboration's standardized case definitions have revolutionized vaccine safety by enabling consistent AEFI identification across diverse settings and populations.

Effective vaccine safety surveillance requires balancing vigilance with perspective, recognizing that vaccines prevent far more harm than they cause while maintaining rigorous monitoring to detect and address legitimate safety concerns. As vaccination programs expand and new vaccines emerge, robust pharmacovigilance systems will remain indispensable for protecting public health and maintaining confidence in immunization.

Future Directions

Brighton Collaboration continues expanding its portfolio of case definitions, addressing emerging vaccines and newly recognized adverse events. The initiative promotes capacity building for proper definition implementation. Integration with electronic health records and automated surveillance systems enhances definition utility.

Vaccine safety surveillance forms a vital shield for public health, powering immunization programs to prevent diseases while swiftly curbing risks - a focus this chapter has explored through the unique challenges of monitoring shots given to healthy people, where distinguishing true adverse events from vaccination failures demands sharp systems and protocols. Adverse Events Following Immunization span minor reactions to serious ones, with WHO's classification guiding responses to product issues, errors, or coincidences, backed by rigorous reporting, investigation, and causality checks. Global teamwork via the WHO Global Advisory Committee, national efforts like India's AEFI system, and Brighton Collaboration's standardized definitions ensure consistent, worldwide vigilance amid controversies. Ultimately, effective surveillance balances alertness with perspective - vaccines save far more lives than they risk - remaining essential as programs grow and new vaccines arrive to sustain trust and protection.

CHAPTER 9

PHARMACOVIGILANCE METHODS

KEY OUTCOMES

Upon completion of this chapter, learners will be able to:

1. Distinguish between passive and active surveillance approaches in pharmacovigilance
2. Describe the structure and function of spontaneous reporting systems
3. Explain the operational principles of sentinel site monitoring
4. Compare different observational study designs for pharmacovigilance research
5. Understand prescription event monitoring methodology and applications
6. Evaluate the strengths and limitations of various surveillance methods
7. Apply appropriate methods for specific drug safety questions
8. Recognize the complementary nature of different pharmacovigilance approaches

ABSTRACT

Pharmacovigilance methods encompass the diverse surveillance techniques and study designs employed to detect, assess, and monitor adverse drug reactions throughout a medicine's lifecycle. This chapter systematically explores the methodological approaches to drug safety monitoring, ranging from passive surveillance systems to active monitoring strategies and formal epidemiological investigations. Each method offers distinct advantages and limitations regarding sensitivity, specificity, resource requirements, and applicability to different safety questions. Passive surveillance through spontaneous reporting systems provides broad coverage and early signal detection capability, while active surveillance offers more complete data capture for targeted monitoring. Observational study designs including case-control and cohort studies enable quantification of adverse event risks and identification of causal relationships. Post-marketing surveillance studies bridge the gap between controlled clinical trials and real-world medication use. Understanding the complementary roles of different pharmacovigilance methods enables construction of comprehensive drug safety monitoring systems. This chapter provides learners with essential knowledge of surveillance methodologies, preparing them to participate in pharmacovigilance activities across clinical, research, and regulatory settings.

9.1 PASSIVE SURVEILLANCE - SPONTANEOUS REPORTING SYSTEMS

Spontaneous reporting systems constitute the cornerstone of global pharmacovigilance, serving as the primary method for detecting unexpected adverse drug reactions in routine clinical practice. These passive surveillance systems rely on voluntary reporting of suspected adverse events by healthcare professionals, patients, and pharmaceutical companies to regulatory authorities.

Definition and Principles

Spontaneous reporting represents passive pharmacovigilance where adverse drug reactions are reported voluntarily without systematic patient enrollment or follow-up. The system captures suspected reactions recognized during routine healthcare delivery. Reports typically include patient information, drug details, reaction description, and reporter information. Unlike active surveillance or formal studies, spontaneous reporting does not require predetermined study protocols or structured data collection beyond basic reporting forms.

System Components

Effective spontaneous reporting systems incorporate several essential elements. **Reporting sources** include healthcare professionals (physicians, pharmacists, nurses), patients and consumers, pharmaceutical manufacturers, and other healthcare institutions. **Reporting mechanisms** provide multiple channels including paper forms, telephone hotlines, online portals, and mobile applications to facilitate easy submission.

National databases maintained by regulatory authorities collect, store, and analyze reports. Major databases include the FDA Adverse Event Reporting System (FAERS) in the United States, the Yellow Card Scheme database in the United Kingdom, the European EudraVigilance system, and VigiBase maintained by the WHO Uppsala Monitoring Centre containing over 20 million reports from 130 countries.

Strengths of Spontaneous Reporting

The primary advantage lies in comprehensive coverage encompassing all marketed drugs, all patient populations, and extended observation periods beyond clinical trial timeframes. This broad coverage enables detection of rare adverse reactions occurring in fewer than 1 in 10,000 patients, events impossible to detect in pre-marketing clinical trials typically involving several thousand subjects.

Low cost compared to active surveillance or formal studies makes spontaneous reporting sustainable for long-term monitoring. Minimal resource requirements allow continuous operation without significant infrastructure investment. The systems generate early signals of potential safety problems, enabling rapid investigation and regulatory action when needed.

Spontaneous reporting captures reactions in diverse populations including children, elderly patients, pregnant women, and patients with comorbidities often excluded from clinical trials. Real-world medication uses patterns, including off label prescribing and drug interactions, are reflected in reports. The systems accommodate any type of adverse reaction regardless of whether previously recognized or completely unexpected.

Limitations and Challenges

Despite substantial benefits, spontaneous reporting has inherent limitations. **Underreporting** represents the most significant weakness, with estimates suggesting only 1-10% of adverse reactions are actually reported. Reporting rates vary by event severity, drug novelty, and reporter awareness. Serious and unexpected reactions receive preferential reporting while common, well-known reactions are underreported.

Incomplete information frequently limits report utility. Missing data regarding patient demographics, concomitant medications, medical history, or outcome details complicates causality assessment. **Reporting bias** affects data quality, with preferential reporting of serious events, reactions to new drugs, or highly publicized adverse effects. Media attention creates temporary reporting spikes that may not reflect true incidence changes.

Inability to calculate incidence rates fundamentally limits spontaneous reporting analysis. Without knowing total exposed populations, absolute risk cannot be determined. Reports provide numerators (adverse event cases) without denominators (total drug exposure), preventing direct risk estimation. Comparative analysis between drugs remains problematic due to differential reporting rates and exposure levels.

Duplicate reports occur when the same event is reported by multiple sources (patient, physician, manufacturer), potentially inflating apparent case numbers. **Causality uncertainty** exists since reports represent suspected rather than confirmed associations, requiring individual assessment.

Data Analysis and Signal Detection

Regulatory authorities employ statistical methods to detect safety signals within spontaneous reporting databases. **Disproportionality analysis** compares observed versus expected reporting rates for specific drug-event combinations. Common metrics include the Proportional Reporting Ratio (PRR), Reporting Odds Ratio (ROR), and Information Component (IC).

These methods identify statistical associations meriting further investigation rather than proving causation. Signals undergo clinical review, additional data collection, and formal epidemiological studies for confirmation. The spontaneous reporting system serves as an early warning system triggering comprehensive safety evaluation rather than providing definitive evidence.

Future Developments

Technological advances enhance spontaneous reporting including electronic health record integration enabling automated adverse event detection and reporting, mobile applications improving patient reporting accessibility, natural language processing extracting relevant information from narrative reports, and machine learning algorithms improving signal detection sensitivity and specificity.

9.2 YELLOW CARD SCHEME

The Yellow Card Scheme represents the United Kingdom's spontaneous adverse drug reaction reporting system, established in 1964 following the thalidomide tragedy. Operating as one of the world's longest-running pharmacovigilance systems, the Yellow Card Scheme has served as a model for spontaneous reporting programs globally.

Historical Background

The thalidomide disaster, where a sedative caused severe birth defects affecting thousands of children, demonstrated the inadequacy of existing drug safety monitoring. The Yellow Card Scheme emerged as a systematic approach to collecting adverse reaction reports from healthcare professionals. The distinctive yellow reporting cards gave the system its name and created memorable branding supporting awareness.

System Structure and Operation

The Yellow Card Scheme is operated by the Medicines and Healthcare products Regulatory Agency (MHRA) in partnership with the Commission on Human Medicines (CHM). The system accepts reports from multiple sources including doctors, dentists, pharmacists, nurses, coroners, and other healthcare professionals. In 2005, the scheme expanded to include patient reporting, recognizing that patients often experience reactions not communicated to healthcare providers.

Reporting Process

Reporters submit yellow cards through various channels including traditional paper forms available in the British National Formulary and medical offices, an online reporting system accessible via the MHRA website, a mobile app enabling convenient submission, and telephone reporting for urgent cases. The reporting form collects essential information including patient age and sex, suspected drug(s) with dose and dates, suspected adverse reaction details, outcome, other medications, relevant medical history, and reporter information.

Reporting Criteria

The scheme encourages reporting based on drug status and reaction type. For established drugs and vaccines, serious or unusual suspected reactions warrant reporting. For new drugs identified by a black triangle symbol, all suspected reactions including minor ones should be reported. The black triangle designation applies to medicines under intensive monitoring, typically for the first two years post-approval.

Data Management

Submitted reports enter a national database where medical reviewers assess causality, duplicate reports are identified and merged, reaction terms are coded using standardized terminology (MedDRA), and serious cases are prioritized for detailed evaluation. The MHRA shares data with the WHO Programme for International Drug Monitoring, contributing to global pharmacovigilance.

Signal Detection and Action

Accumulated Yellow Card data undergoes regular analysis to detect safety signals. Statistical methods identify unusual reporting patterns. Detected signals trigger further investigation including targeted active surveillance, observational studies, review of international data, and manufacturer investigations. Confirmed safety concerns lead to regulatory actions such as label updates, restriction of indications, Dear Healthcare Professional communications, or in severe cases, market withdrawal.

Impact and Examples

The Yellow Card Scheme has successfully identified numerous adverse reactions including oculomucocutaneous syndrome with practolol (leading to withdrawal), rare blood dyscrasias with various medicines, Stevens-Johnson syndrome with multiple drugs, and hepatotoxicity with numerous agents. Patient reporting has particularly enhanced detection of reactions to over-the-counter medicines and vaccines.

Public Awareness Initiatives

The MHRA conducts public awareness campaigns educating healthcare professionals about reporting importance, informing patients about their reporting rights, highlighting specific therapeutic areas requiring enhanced surveillance, and publishing annual reports summarizing scheme activities and findings. The yellow card symbol has become widely recognized, reinforcing the scheme's public health role.

Table 16: Yellow Card Scheme Workflow

Stage	Process Component	Outcome
Report Submission	Healthcare professionals or patients submit suspected ADR via multiple channels	Yellow card received by MHRA
Initial Assessment	Medical reviewers evaluate report completeness and seriousness	Report entered into database, follow-up requested if needed
Signal Detection	Statistical analysis identifies unusual reporting patterns	Potential safety signals flagged
Investigation	Detailed evaluation of signals through additional data collection	Confirmed or refuted safety concerns
Regulatory Action	Implementation of risk minimization measures	Label updates, restrictions, or withdrawals

9.3 CASE SERIES ANALYSIS

Case series analysis represents a descriptive pharmacovigilance method examining multiple individual cases of a suspected adverse drug reaction to identify patterns, characteristics, and potential causal relationships. While lacking the comparative structure of formal epidemiological studies, case series provide valuable insights particularly for rare reactions or newly marketed drugs.

Methodology

Case series analysis involves systematic collection and examination of individual case reports sharing common features such as exposure to the same drug, occurrence of the same adverse event, or occurrence within a defined population or timeframe. Researchers compile detailed information from each case including patient demographics, drug exposure details (dose, duration, timing), clinical manifestations of the adverse event, temporal relationships, outcomes, and alternative explanations.

The analysis identifies common patterns across cases, examines dose-response relationships, evaluates temporal associations between drug exposure and event onset, assesses dechallenge and rechallenge experiences, and reviews biological plausibility. Unlike spontaneous reports that may contain incomplete information, case series typically involve detailed case descriptions with comprehensive clinical data.

Applications in Pharmacovigilance

Case series serve multiple purposes within pharmacovigilance frameworks. They provide initial evidence of potential adverse drug reactions when individual cases accumulate suggesting a pattern. Early recognition of unexpected reactions often begins with astute clinicians noting similar events in patients receiving the same medication. Published case series alert the medical community to potential safety concerns warranting vigilance.

For rare reactions occurring infrequently, case series may represent the only feasible method to study the phenomenon. Controlled studies become impractical when events affect fewer than 1 in 100,000 patients. Detailed case descriptions enable characterization of reaction features including typical presentation, time course, severity, and predisposing factors. This characterization aids clinical recognition and management.

Strengths and Limitations

Case series offer several advantages including relatively simple methodology not requiring complex study designs, ability to describe rare events that formal studies cannot feasibly investigate, detailed clinical information providing insights into reaction mechanisms and risk factors, and rapid publication alerting healthcare providers to emerging safety concerns.

However, significant limitations constrain case series interpretation. The absence of control groups prevents determination of whether event rates exceed background incidence. Selection bias affects case identification, as published series may preferentially include severe or unusual cases. Confounding variables including concurrent medications, underlying diseases, and patient characteristics cannot be adequately controlled. Causality assessment remains uncertain without comparative data demonstrating increased risk with drug exposure versus non-exposure.

Published Case Series Examples

Historical examples demonstrate case series impact on pharmacovigilance. Early reports of practolol-induced oculomucocutaneous syndrome emerged through case series descriptions. Eosinophilia-myalgia syndrome associated with L-tryptophan was first recognized through case series. Hepatotoxicity patterns with various drugs have been characterized through detailed case compilations.

Role in Signal Generation

Case series function as important signal generation tools within comprehensive pharmacovigilance systems. When spontaneous reports suggest a potential safety issue, detailed case series analysis provides deeper understanding. The systematic examination may reveal characteristic features supporting causation, identify subpopulations at particular risk, or suggest mechanisms underlying the adverse reaction. These insights guide subsequent formal epidemiological investigations confirming or refuting suspected associations.

9.4 STIMULATED REPORTING METHODS

Stimulated reporting represents an intermediate approach between purely passive spontaneous reporting and fully active surveillance, involving systematic efforts to increase reporting rates for specific drugs, events, or populations. This method enhances passive surveillance sensitivity during periods when heightened vigilance is warranted.

Principles and Rationale

Standard spontaneous reporting suffers from underreporting, with many adverse reactions never reaching regulatory authorities. Stimulated reporting addresses this limitation through targeted interventions increasing healthcare provider awareness and reporting motivation. The approach maintains spontaneous reporting's broad coverage while improving sensitivity for priority safety questions.

Stimulation Strategies

Various methods stimulate enhanced reporting. **Educational interventions** include targeted communications to healthcare professionals highlighting specific drugs requiring intensive monitoring, providing education about adverse events of concern, distributing reporting forms directly to relevant specialists, and conducting training sessions on adverse reaction recognition and reporting.

Reminder systems implement regular prompts encouraging reporting such as inclusion of reporting information in prescription systems, periodic mailings or emails to healthcare providers, and point-of-care reminders in electronic health records. **Focused campaigns** may target new drug launches with intensive monitoring during initial post-marketing periods, specific therapeutic areas where safety concerns have emerged, or patient populations requiring special attention.

Pharmacist-based initiatives leverage community pharmacy networks by educating pharmacists about targeted drugs or reactions, providing simplified reporting mechanisms, and establishing liaison between pharmacies and regulatory authorities. **Patient involvement** through direct-to-patient educational materials informing about specific reactions and simplified patient reporting systems specifically for targeted drugs.

Applications

Stimulated reporting proves particularly valuable in several scenarios. During new drug introductions, enhanced surveillance detects unexpected reactions in real-world use. When post-marketing studies identify potential signals, stimulated reporting increases case ascertainment enabling better risk characterization. For drugs with known serious but rare reactions, ongoing stimulated reporting maintains surveillance. Special populations including pediatric or geriatric patients may benefit from targeted reporting enhancement.

Effectiveness and Limitations

Evidence demonstrates that stimulated reporting substantially increases reporting rates compared to standard passive surveillance. Studies show interventions can increase reporting by 2 to 10-fold during active stimulation periods. However, effects may be temporary, with reporting declining after intervention cessation. The approach requires ongoing resource investment for sustained impact.

Stimulated reporting cannot completely eliminate underreporting bias. Selective enhancement may create artificial differences in reporting rates between monitored and non-monitored drugs, complicating comparative analysis. The method works best as a temporary intensification strategy during critical monitoring periods rather than long-term surveillance approach.

9.5 ACTIVE SURVEILLANCE SYSTEMS

Active surveillance represents proactive pharmacovigilance where systematic, organized data collection occurs through predetermined protocols rather than relying on spontaneous reporting. This approach provides more complete and reliable safety information though requiring greater resources than passive systems.

Defining Characteristics

Active surveillance involves systematic identification of exposed populations, regular contact with patients or healthcare providers to ascertain adverse events, standardized data collection procedures, and predetermined follow-up schedules. Unlike passive systems awaiting reports, active surveillance proactively seeks adverse event information from defined cohorts. The methodology resembles prospective cohort studies but typically operates within healthcare delivery systems rather than research-specific frameworks.

Types of Active Surveillance

Several active surveillance approaches exist with varying intensity and scope. **Registry-based surveillance** establishes disease or drug registries systematically following patients exposed to specific medications or experiencing particular conditions. Registries collect comprehensive data including detailed patient characteristics, drug exposure information, clinical outcomes, and long-term follow-up.

Electronic health record surveillance utilizes automated systems mining electronic medical records to identify adverse events. Algorithms detect specific diagnoses, laboratory abnormalities, or clinical scenarios potentially representing adverse reactions. This approach leverages existing healthcare data infrastructure without requiring additional data collection efforts.

Claims database surveillance analyzes administrative healthcare databases containing insurance claims, hospital discharge records, and pharmacy dispensing information. Large population coverage enables detection of relatively rare events. Linked databases allow assessment of temporal relationships between prescriptions and medical encounters potentially representing adverse events.

Advantages Over Passive Surveillance

Active surveillance offers multiple benefits. **Complete case ascertainment** within monitored populations eliminates underreporting bias affecting spontaneous systems. Known denominators enable calculation of true incidence rates and absolute risk estimates. **Standardized data collection** ensures consistent, comprehensive information facilitating causality assessment. **Prospective design** allows real-time monitoring with immediate response to emerging safety signals.

The ability to calculate incidence rates represents a fundamental advantage, enabling direct risk quantification rather than relying on disproportionality analysis. Comparative risk assessment across different drugs becomes feasible with known exposure populations. Statistical power for rare event detection increases through large population coverage.

Limitations and Challenges

Despite advantages, active surveillance faces constraints. **High resource requirements** including personnel, technology infrastructure, and ongoing operational costs limit feasibility for universal application. Systems typically monitor selected drugs, specific populations, or adverse events rather than providing comprehensive coverage.

Delayed implementation occurs as active surveillance systems require time to establish, often missing early post-marketing periods. Data privacy regulations complicate access to healthcare information necessary for surveillance. Technical challenges include developing accurate event detection algorithms, managing false positive signals, and integrating diverse data sources.

Active surveillance may miss events occurring outside monitored healthcare systems or populations. The approach works optimally for serious adverse events leading to medical encounters captured in healthcare databases but may fail to detect events not resulting in healthcare utilization.

Implementation Examples

Several large-scale active surveillance systems demonstrate feasibility and value. The Sentinel Initiative in the United States monitors drug safety using distributed data networks accessing over 200 million individuals' healthcare data. The European Union ADR system integrates multiple national databases for coordinated surveillance. The Clinical Practice Research Datalink (CPRD) in the United Kingdom provides longitudinal primary care data for pharmacovigilance research.

Table 17: Comparison of Passive and Active Surveillance

Characteristic	Passive Surveillance	Active Surveillance
Data Collection	Voluntary reporting	Systematic ascertainment
Population Coverage	All patients, all drugs	Defined populations, selected drugs
Completeness	Significant underreporting	High case ascertainment
Incidence Calculation	Not possible	Feasible with known denominators

Resource Requirements	Low	High
Response Time	Rapid signal generation	May have implementation delays

9.6 SENTINEL SITES FOR DRUG MONITORING

Sentinel site surveillance establishes designated healthcare facilities that conduct enhanced pharmacovigilance activities, serving as early warning systems for adverse drug reactions within broader surveillance networks. This targeted approach concentrates resources at selected sites while maintaining population representativeness.

Concept and Structure

Sentinel sites are healthcare facilities selected to conduct intensive drug safety monitoring, reporting adverse reactions more completely and rapidly than general healthcare settings. Sites typically include major hospitals, specialized clinics, or healthcare systems with adequate infrastructure and trained personnel. The network of sentinel sites provides population coverage representing diverse geographic regions, demographic groups, and clinical settings.

Selection criteria emphasize facilities with established pharmacovigilance expertise, robust patient populations for adequate event capture, electronic health record systems facilitating data collection, specialized clinical services relevant to monitored drugs, and commitment to surveillance participation. A manageable number of sentinel sites balances comprehensive coverage with feasibility of intensive monitoring.

Operational Framework

Sentinel sites implement standardized protocols for adverse event detection, documentation, and reporting. Dedicated pharmacovigilance staff coordinate activities including routine review of patient records, active solicitation of adverse event reports from clinicians, validation and documentation of suspected reactions, and timely transmission to national databases. Regular training ensures consistent application of protocols across sites.

The approach combines elements of passive and active surveillance. Within sentinel sites, active methods identify adverse events through systematic review while maintaining spontaneous reporting from healthcare providers. This hybrid approach captures more complete data than purely passive systems while remaining more feasible than comprehensive active surveillance.

Priority Setting

Sentinel surveillance typically focuses on specific monitoring priorities rather than attempting comprehensive coverage of all drugs and events. Priorities may include newly approved drugs requiring intensive post-marketing monitoring, drugs with known serious adverse reactions requiring ongoing vigilance, therapeutic areas with high safety concerns, or special populations including hospitalized patients where serious reactions commonly occur.

Advantages

The sentinel site approach offers multiple benefits. Concentrated resources at designated facilities enable intensive monitoring not feasible system wide. Trained personnel with pharmacovigilance expertise improve adverse event recognition and reporting quality. Standardized protocols ensure data consistency. The network structure provides broader population coverage than single-center studies while maintaining feasibility.

Sentinel sites can respond rapidly to emerging safety questions, implementing targeted surveillance protocols quickly. The established infrastructure enables efficient conduct of focused investigations when regulatory authorities require additional data about specific safety concerns.

Challenges

Representativeness concerns arise as sentinel site populations may not reflect broader population characteristics. Urban academic medical centers often serve as sentinel sites, potentially missing adverse events occurring primarily in rural or community settings. Sicker, hospitalized populations at sentinel sites may experience different adverse event profiles than outpatients.

Resource intensity remains substantial despite being less than comprehensive active surveillance. Sites require dedicated staff, training, and infrastructure. Sustainability depends on continued funding and institutional commitment. Data quality may vary across sites despite standardization efforts.

Applications

Sentinel sites function effectively for monitoring drugs used primarily in hospital settings, post-marketing commitments for new drug approvals, surveillance during public health emergencies, and targeted investigation of specific safety signals. The approach proves particularly valuable when comprehensive population surveillance is unnecessary or infeasible but enhanced monitoring beyond spontaneous reporting is warranted.

9.7 DRUG EVENT MONITORING AND REGISTRIES

Drug event monitoring and registry-based surveillance represent systematic approaches following defined patient cohorts exposed to medications, collecting comprehensive safety data through standardized protocols. These methods bridge passive and active surveillance, providing detailed long-term safety information.

Registry Definitions

A drug registry is an organized system collecting uniform data on patients exposed to specific medications to evaluate specified outcomes. Registries prospectively follow exposed cohorts, capturing adverse events, effectiveness outcomes, and other relevant clinical information. Unlike spontaneous reporting capturing individual cases, registries systematically enroll and monitor patient populations.

Disease registries similarly track patients with specific conditions, potentially including medication exposures and outcomes. Both registry types contribute to pharmacovigilance through systematic data collection enabling incidence rate calculation and risk factor identification.

Registry Types and Purposes

Product registries focus on patients receiving medications, especially drugs with significant safety concerns or requiring specialized monitoring. These registries may be mandated as post-marketing commitments for drug approval. Examples include registries for clozapine monitoring agranulocytosis risk, isotretinoin registries preventing pregnancy exposure, and thalidomide distribution programs with strict safety protocols.

Pregnancy registries specifically monitor medication exposures during pregnancy, assessing teratogenic risks and maternal-fetal outcomes. These registries address critical knowledge gaps as pregnant women are typically excluded from clinical trials. Data collection includes pregnancy outcomes, birth defects, maternal complications, and infant development.

Disease registries for conditions like cancer, rheumatoid arthritis, or multiple sclerosis track medication exposures, disease progression, and outcomes within specific patient populations. These registries enable evaluation of drug safety and effectiveness in real-world clinical contexts.

Data Collection Methods

Registry data come from multiple sources including healthcare provider reporting through standardized forms, patient self-reporting via questionnaires or diaries, medical record review by registry staff, and linkage with electronic health records or administrative databases. Comprehensive registries employ multiple data sources for complete capture.

Follow-up protocols specify regular intervals for data collection, often including baseline assessment at enrollment, periodic follow-up during treatment, and long-term surveillance after treatment discontinuation. Active follow-up through phone calls, clinic visits, or surveys maintains patient engagement.

Advantages

Registries provide numerous benefits for pharmacovigilance. Systematic enrollment and follow-up yield more complete data than spontaneous reporting. Known exposed populations enable incidence rate calculation. Detailed clinical information supports causality assessment. Prospective design captures events as they occur rather than relying on retrospective recall.

Registries can detect long-term effects appearing months or years after exposure, timeframes poorly captured by spontaneous reporting. Subgroup analyses identify populations at particular risk. Comparative analyses may assess outcomes across different treatments within disease registries.

Challenges and Limitations

Registry operation requires substantial resources including infrastructure for patient enrollment, data collection systems, personnel for data management, and long-term funding for sustained operation.

Patient recruitment and retention pose ongoing challenges. Selection bias may occur if enrolled patients differ systematically from those declining participation.

Incomplete follow-up reduces data quality and may bias results if patients experiencing adverse events discontinue participation. Causality assessment remains challenging as registries typically lack unexposed control groups. Confounding by indication occurs when disease severity influences treatment selection and outcomes.

Regulatory Applications

Regulatory authorities increasingly mandate registries as conditions for drug approval, particularly for medications with serious known risks. Risk Evaluation and Mitigation Strategies (REMS) in the United States may include registry requirements. European Medicines Agency Risk Management Plans similarly incorporate registry-based surveillance.

Registry data support regulatory decision-making regarding label updates, indication restrictions, or safety communications. Evidence from registries has influenced important regulatory actions for numerous medications.

9.8 PRESCRIPTION EVENT MONITORING (PEM)

Prescription Event Monitoring represents a specialized form of cohort event monitoring conducted in the United Kingdom by the Drug Safety Research Unit. PEM provides systematic post-marketing surveillance for newly licensed medications through observational cohort studies using prescription and outcome data.

Methodology

PEM studies begin shortly after drug launch, identifying patients prescribed the new medication through pharmacy dispensing records or prescription data. The Drug Safety Research Unit obtains prescribing information from the National Health Service, identifying general practitioners who prescribed the drug. Participating physicians receive questionnaires requesting information about patients receiving prescriptions including indication for use, patient demographics, medical history, concurrent medications, clinical events occurring after drug initiation, outcomes, and treatment duration.

The observational design follows patients in routine clinical practice without intervention. All events occurring after drug initiation are captured regardless of suspected causality, termed "events" rather than "adverse reactions" to avoid presuming causation. Follow-up typically extends for defined periods, commonly six months to one year after first prescription.

Analysis Approaches

PEM studies calculate incidence rates for various clinical events within the monitored cohort. Temporal analysis examines event timing relative to treatment initiation, with clustering shortly after treatment start suggesting potential drug causation. Dose-response relationships provide additional causality evidence.

Comparisons with expected background rates in general populations help identify elevated event incidences. Some studies include comparison cohorts receiving alternative treatments for similar indications, though most PEM studies analyze single drug cohorts. Serious events receive detailed investigation including medical record review and causality assessment.

Strengths

PEM provides valuable early post-marketing safety data for new drugs. Large patient numbers, typically 10,000 or more per study, enable detection of relatively uncommon adverse events. Real-world prescribing patterns reflect actual clinical practice including off label uses and diverse patient populations. Capture of all events, not just those suspected as adverse reactions, reduces reporting bias.

The systematic approach generates more complete data than spontaneous reporting during critical early post-marketing periods. Incidence rate calculation provides quantitative risk estimates. The method has proven feasible for sustainable operation monitoring numerous new drugs.

Limitations

PEM faces several constraints. Reliance on physician reporting introduces potential underascertainment despite systematic solicitation. Questionnaire-based data collection limits detail compared to comprehensive medical record review. Lack of unexposed control groups complicates attribution of causality. Confounding by indication affects interpretation as prescribing patterns relate to patient characteristics and disease severity.

The approach captures events leading to medical attention or recognized by physicians but may miss mild reactions not prompting healthcare encounters. Follow-up period limitations mean long-term adverse effects may not be detected. Resource requirements restrict the number of drugs simultaneously monitored.

Applications and Impact

PEM has contributed significantly to identifying important adverse reactions for numerous newly marketed drugs. Studies have detected previously unrecognized safety signals, characterized event incidence and risk factors, and provided evidence supporting or refuting suspected associations. Findings have informed regulatory decisions and product labeling updates.

The PEM model has influenced development of similar cohort event monitoring approaches in other countries. The methodology demonstrates feasibility of systematic early post-marketing surveillance bridging the gap between pre-approval clinical trials and long-term spontaneous reporting.

9.9 COMPARATIVE OBSERVATIONAL STUDIES

Comparative observational studies represent epidemiological investigations comparing adverse event rates between patient groups with different drug exposures, providing quantitative risk estimates and enabling causal inference. Unlike spontaneous reporting or single-cohort surveillance, comparative studies incorporate control groups allowing determination of whether event rates exceed background incidence.

Fundamental Principles

Observational studies examine naturally occurring exposures rather than assigning treatments through randomization. Investigators identify patient populations with different medication exposures, ascertain outcomes, and compare event rates between groups. The comparative design controls for background disease incidence, enabling attribution of excess events to drug exposure.

Multiple study designs serve comparative purposes, each with characteristic strengths and limitations. Selection of appropriate design depends on the research question, outcome frequency, available data sources, and resource constraints. Common designs include cross-sectional studies, case-control studies, and cohort studies.

Study Design Selection Considerations

Design choice depends on several factors. **Outcome frequency** influences feasibility, with rare events better studied through case-control designs while common outcomes suit cohort approaches. **Temporal relationships** determine whether prospective or retrospective designs are appropriate. **Data availability** constrains feasible approaches, as some designs require extensive historical data while others need ongoing data collection.

Resource constraints affect design selection, with nested case-control studies offering efficiency advantages over full cohort analyses when outcomes are rare. Research objectives guide design choice, as some questions require prospective follow-up while others can be addressed retrospectively.

Role in Pharmacovigilance

Comparative observational studies serve critical roles within pharmacovigilance frameworks. Following signal detection through spontaneous reporting, formal epidemiological studies test hypotheses and quantify risks. Regulatory authorities increasingly require comparative post-marketing studies as conditions for drug approval or in response to safety concerns.

These studies provide risk estimates needed for informed prescribing decisions and risk-benefit assessments. Evidence from well-designed observational studies influences regulatory actions including label changes, restriction of indications, or market withdrawals. The studies also identify risk factors and susceptible populations requiring special precautions.

Methodological Challenges

Observational studies face inherent challenges distinguishing them from randomized controlled trials. **Confounding by indication** occurs when factors influencing treatment selection also affect outcome risk. Patients receiving different medications may differ systematically in ways affecting adverse event risk independent of drug effects.

Selection bias arises from non-random exposure assignment. Channeling occurs when drugs are preferentially prescribed to particular patient subgroups. **Information bias** results from differential outcome ascertainment between exposure groups. **Unmeasured confounding** represents perhaps the greatest limitation, as unknown or unmeasurable factors may explain apparent associations.

Statistical methods address some biases through multivariable adjustment, propensity score matching, or instrumental variable approaches, but residual confounding remains possible. Sensitivity analyses explore robustness of findings to unmeasured confounding. Despite limitations, well-designed observational studies provide valuable causal evidence, particularly when biological plausibility, dose-response relationships, and consistency across studies support associations

9.10 CROSS-SECTIONAL STUDIES

Cross-sectional studies examine exposure and outcome simultaneously within defined populations at single time points, providing snapshots of drug use patterns and associated adverse events. While less commonly employed for pharmacovigilance than cohort or case-control designs, cross-sectional studies serve specific purposes in drug safety assessment.

Design Characteristics

Cross-sectional studies assess both exposure (drug use) and outcome (adverse event) simultaneously without following subjects over time. Investigators survey defined populations, collecting data on medication use and presence of adverse events at the time of assessment. The temporal relationship between exposure and outcome may be uncertain as both are measured concurrently.

Survey-based cross-sectional studies administer questionnaires to population samples ascertaining medication use, health outcomes, and relevant characteristics. Database cross-sectional analyses query healthcare databases at defined time points, identifying patients with drug exposures and concurrent diagnoses potentially representing adverse events.

Applications in Pharmacovigilance

Cross-sectional studies serve several pharmacovigilance purposes. **Prevalence estimation** of adverse reactions within treated populations provides important safety information. Studies can describe patterns of drug use including off-label prescribing, polypharmacy, and adherence issues potentially affecting safety.

Hypothesis generation occurs through identification of associations meriting further investigation with more definitive study designs. Cross-sectional studies enable rapid assessment of safety questions when time constraints preclude longitudinal study conduct. Pharmacoepidemiological surveys characterize drug utilization patterns and associated outcomes in specific populations or healthcare settings.

Advantages

Cross-sectional studies offer practical advantages including relatively simple and economical design compared to longitudinal studies, feasibility of rapid completion as no follow-up period is required, and ability to examine multiple exposures and outcomes simultaneously. Large population surveys efficiently collect data on numerous health issues and medication uses.

For prevalent conditions persisting over time, cross-sectional designs effectively capture associations. The approach works well for descriptive objectives characterizing patterns without requiring causal inference.

Limitations

Fundamental limitations restrict cross-sectional study utility for causal inference. **Temporal ambiguity** prevents determination of whether exposure preceded outcome or vice versa. For acute adverse reactions, uncertainty about whether the medication was initiated before or after symptom onset complicates interpretation. The design captures prevalent rather than incident cases, potentially missing acute reactions resolving rapidly.

Reverse causation may occur when outcomes influence exposure rather than the reverse. For example, finding higher medication use among patients with certain symptoms may reflect treatment of those symptoms rather than drug-induced effects. **Survivor bias** affects studies of serious adverse events as patients experiencing fatal or severely disabling reactions are absent from surveyed populations.

The cross-sectional approach cannot assess temporal relationships like effect persistence after treatment cessation or latency periods between exposure and outcome. Establishing dose-response relationships proves difficult without longitudinal exposure data.

Appropriate Use

Cross-sectional studies function best as preliminary investigations suggesting hypotheses for testing through longitudinal designs. They effectively describe prevalence of known adverse reactions, characterize drug use patterns in populations, and provide rapid initial assessment of urgent safety questions. However, causal conclusions require confirmation through cohort or case-control studies establishing appropriate temporal sequences.

9.11 CASE-CONTROL STUDIES

Case-control studies represent efficient designs for investigating rare adverse drug reactions by comparing medication exposures between patients experiencing adverse events (cases) and similar patients without the events (controls). This retrospective approach offers advantages for studying uncommon outcomes.

Design Fundamentals

Case-control studies begin by identifying cases—patients with the adverse event of interest. Controls are selected from the source population that gave rise to the cases, representing individuals at risk for the event. Investigators then look backward in time, comparing medication exposures between cases and controls. Exposure differences indicate associations between drugs and adverse outcomes.

The design proves particularly efficient for rare outcomes because case identification comes first, avoiding need to follow large cohorts to observe sufficient events. For example, investigating a serious adverse reaction occurring in 1 per 10,000 patients would require cohort follow-up of enormous populations. Case-control studies instead identify affected patients and efficiently compare their exposures to controls.

Case Definition and Selection

Rigorous case definition ensures valid results. Cases should meet explicit diagnostic criteria established a priori, with objective verification through medical records, laboratory tests, or expert review reducing misclassification. Incident (newly occurring) cases generally provide clearer results than prevalent cases as exposure status is more certain.

Case sources include hospitals where serious reactions present, disease registries systematically documenting specific conditions, healthcare databases with diagnostic codes, or spontaneous reporting systems where detailed case investigation occurs. Regardless of source, complete case ascertainment within defined populations strengthens inferences.

Control Selection

Control selection represents the most critical design element affecting validity. Controls should represent the source population from which cases arose, with similar opportunity for drug exposure and event ascertainment. If cases come from a hospital, appropriate controls might include patients hospitalized for unrelated conditions.

Multiple control selection strategies exist. **Population-based controls** represent the general population using random digit dialing, voter registration lists, or population registries. **Hospital controls** include patients hospitalized for conditions unrelated to the study drug. **Nested case-control** designs select controls from cohorts already under surveillance. Multiple controls per case increase statistical power for rare exposures.

Analysis and Interpretation

Case-control studies calculate the **odds ratio (OR)**, representing the odds of exposure among cases relative to controls. An OR greater than 1 suggests increased risk with exposure, while OR less than 1 indicates protective effects. Statistical methods adjust for potential confounders including age, sex, comorbidities, and other risk factors.

Advantages and Limitations

The primary advantage is efficiency for rare outcomes, requiring smaller sample sizes than cohort studies. Retrospective data collection provides rapid results. Multiple exposures can be examined simultaneously. However, recall bias may occur if cases remember exposures differently than controls. Selection bias affects results if controls inadequately represent the source population. Temporal relationships may be unclear, and unmeasured confounding remains possible.

9.12 COHORT STUDIES

Cohort studies follow groups of patients forward in time, comparing adverse event rates between exposed and unexposed populations. This prospective approach provides strong causal evidence for pharmacovigilance investigations.

Design Principles

Cohort studies identify patients based on exposure status—those receiving the drug of interest (exposed cohort) and those not receiving it (unexposed cohort). Both groups are followed over time to ascertain adverse events. Comparison of event rates between cohorts determines whether drug exposure increases risk.

Prospective cohorts enroll patients and follow them forward from the present. Retrospective cohorts identify historical exposures and trace outcomes through existing records. Both designs maintain the essential feature of determining exposure before outcome occurrence.

Exposure Definition

Clear exposure classification is essential. Exposed patients are those initiating the study drug during the enrollment period. Comparison groups may include unexposed patients, those receiving alternative medications, or patients before drug availability. Multiple exposure levels enable dose-response analysis strengthening causal inference.

Outcome Ascertainment

Systematic follow-up identifies adverse events through regular patient contact, medical record review, healthcare database queries, or linkage with mortality registries. Standardized outcome definitions ensure consistent ascertainment across exposure groups. Blinded outcome assessment reduces detection bias.

Analysis Methods

Cohort studies calculate **relative risk (RR)** or **rate ratios** comparing event rates between exposed and unexposed groups. RR greater than 1 indicates increased risk with exposure. **Attributable risk** quantifies excess events caused by exposure. Multivariable models adjust for confounders.

Advantages

Cohort studies directly measure incidence rates, calculate multiple outcomes simultaneously, establish clear temporal sequences, and minimize recall bias. The design suits common outcomes and enables evaluation of multiple effects from single exposures.

Limitations

Large sample sizes are required for rare outcomes. Prospective cohorts need extended follow-up periods with associated costs. Loss to follow-up may bias results. Confounding by indication remains challenging despite statistical adjustment.

9.13 TARGETED CLINICAL INVESTIGATIONS

Targeted clinical investigations represent focused studies addressing specific safety questions identified through surveillance systems. These investigations may employ various methodologies tailored to the research question.

Purpose and Initiation

When spontaneous reporting or observational studies identify potential safety signals, targeted investigations provide definitive evidence. Regulatory authorities may mandate these studies as post-marketing commitments. The focused nature allows efficient resource allocation to priority safety concerns.

Study Designs

Investigations may utilize randomized controlled trials when ethical, providing highest quality causal evidence. Observational studies serve when randomization is inappropriate. Mechanistic studies explore biological mechanisms underlying adverse reactions. Pharmacokinetic studies examine drug interactions or special population pharmacology.

Implementation

Rapid protocol development and approval enable timely investigation of urgent safety questions. Collaboration between manufacturers, regulators, and academic researchers facilitates efficient conduct. Results inform regulatory decisions and risk management strategies.

9.14 POST-MARKETING SURVEILLANCE STUDIES

Post-marketing surveillance studies encompass diverse methodologies monitoring drug safety after regulatory approval, bridging the gap between pre-approval clinical trials and long-term real-world use.

Phase IV Studies

Post-marketing clinical trials evaluate long-term safety, effectiveness in broader populations, and optimal use conditions. Manufacturers may voluntarily conduct these studies or perform them as post-approval commitments.

Large Simple Trials

These pragmatic trials embedded in clinical practice enroll large populations with minimal inclusion criteria, capturing real-world effectiveness and safety. Simplified data collection reduces costs while maintaining adequate sample sizes.

Database Studies

Administrative databases, electronic health records, and claims data enable large-scale safety monitoring. Automated algorithms detect adverse events efficiently. Linkage between prescription and outcome databases facilitates exposure-outcome assessment.

Risk Management Programs

Structured programs minimize known risks through restricted distribution, mandatory monitoring, or patient education. Registry-based systems ensure appropriate use and monitor outcomes.

Meta-Analysis and Systematic Reviews

Pooling data from multiple studies increases power for rare event detection and provides comprehensive safety assessments across diverse populations.

Pharmacovigilance methods encompass diverse surveillance approaches, each contributing uniquely to comprehensive drug safety monitoring. Passive surveillance through spontaneous reporting provides broad coverage and early signal detection, while active surveillance enables precise risk quantification. Observational study designs ranging from case-control to cohort studies facilitate causal inference and risk factor identification. The complementary nature of these methods necessitates integrated surveillance systems employing multiple approaches.

Effective pharmacovigilance requires selecting appropriate methods for specific safety questions, recognizing each method's strengths and limitations, and synthesizing evidence from multiple sources. As healthcare systems evolve and data resources expand, pharmacovigilance methods continue advancing through electronic health record integration, automated signal detection, and real-world evidence generation. Understanding these methodological foundations prepares practitioners to participate effectively in drug safety monitoring across clinical, regulatory, and public health settings, ultimately protecting patient welfare while enabling beneficial medication use.

CHAPTER 10

COMMUNICATION IN PHARMACOVIGILANCE

KEY OUTCOMES

Upon completion of this chapter, learners will be able to:

1. Understand fundamental principles of effective communication in pharmacovigilance
2. Develop risk communication strategies appropriate for diverse audiences
3. Implement crisis management protocols during drug safety emergencies
4. Communicate effectively with regulatory agencies and business partners
5. Design educational communications for healthcare professionals
6. Conduct appropriate media engagement and public awareness campaigns
7. Prepare Dear Healthcare Professional Communications following regulatory standards
8. Implement risk minimization measures through structured communication approaches

ABSTRACT

Effective communication represents a fundamental pillar of pharmacovigilance, ensuring that drug safety information reaches relevant stakeholders in timely, accurate, and actionable formats. This chapter explores the principles and practices of communication within pharmacovigilance systems, encompassing risk communication strategies, crisis management, regulatory reporting, stakeholder engagement, and public awareness initiatives. Communication in pharmacovigilance serves multiple critical functions including informing prescribing decisions, supporting regulatory actions, maintaining public trust, and facilitating appropriate medication use. The complexity of communicating uncertain, evolving safety information to diverse audiences with varying levels of scientific literacy presents ongoing challenges. This chapter examines structured approaches to developing communication strategies, managing drug safety crises, engaging with regulatory authorities, collaborating with business partners, educating healthcare professionals, and conducting media outreach. Special emphasis is placed on Dear Healthcare Professional Communications and risk minimization measures as practical tools for conveying safety information. Understanding communication principles and practices enables pharmacovigilance professionals to contribute effectively to protecting public health through appropriate information dissemination.

10.1 PRINCIPLES OF EFFECTIVE COMMUNICATION IN PHARMACOVIGILANCE

Effective communication in pharmacovigilance requires adherence to fundamental principles ensuring that safety information achieves intended objectives without causing unintended harm. The unique characteristics of drug safety information - often uncertain, evolving, and potentially alarming - create special communication challenges.

Core Principles

Accuracy represents the foundation of pharmacovigilance communication. All information must be factually correct, scientifically sound, and appropriately contextualized. Misrepresentation of risks or benefits undermines trust and may result in inappropriate treatment decisions. Evidence-based communication relies on systematic evaluation of available data, acknowledging uncertainty when present.

Timeliness ensures safety information reaches stakeholders when needed for decision-making. Delays in communicating serious risks may result in preventable adverse events. However, premature communication of unconfirmed signals may cause unnecessary alarm. Balancing these concerns requires judgment based on signal strength, severity, and availability of alternatives.

Clarity demands that messages be understandable to intended audiences. Technical jargon should be avoided or explained. Complex information requires simplification without sacrificing accuracy. Visual aids, examples, and structured formats enhance comprehension.

Consistency across different communication channels prevents confusion and maintains credibility. Contradictory messages from different sources erode trust. Coordinated communication between regulatory authorities, manufacturers, and professional organizations ensures unified messaging.

Completeness means providing sufficient context for informed decision-making. Risk information should include absolute and relative risks, comparisons with alternative treatments, and implications for practice. Incomplete information may lead to misinterpretation.

Transparency involves openly acknowledging uncertainties, limitations, and knowledge gaps. Honest communication about what is known and unknown maintains credibility and realistic expectations. Hidden information, when later revealed, damages trust far more than initial transparency would have.

Audience Appropriateness

Different stakeholders require tailored communication approaches. **Healthcare professionals** need detailed clinical information, mechanisms of action, risk factors, and management recommendations. Scientific terminology is appropriate with this audience.

Patients and the public require simplified explanations avoiding technical language. Practical implications for medication use, symptom recognition, and when to seek medical attention take priority. Emotional aspects deserve attention as safety information may cause anxiety.

Regulatory authorities expect standardized formats, comprehensive data, and compliance with reporting requirements. Formal, structured communication following established guidelines is essential.

Media requires concise, newsworthy information with clear public health implications. Media communications must anticipate potential misinterpretation and provide context preventing sensationalism.

Communication Objectives

Pharmacovigilance communication serves multiple objectives including informing prescribing and dispensing decisions, supporting regulatory actions, maintaining appropriate medication use, preventing adverse events through risk minimization, enabling informed patient consent, maintaining public trust in medicines regulation, and facilitating reporting of suspected adverse reactions.

Clear identification of communication objectives guides message development. Different objectives may require different approaches, formats, and channels.

Challenges

Communicating uncertainty without undermining necessary confidence in medications poses ongoing challenges. Pharmacovigilance often operates with incomplete data and evolving understanding.

Conveying this uncertainty honestly while maintaining appropriate medication use requires careful balance.

Risk perception differences complicate communication. People often overestimate rare but dramatic risks while underestimating common risks. Framing effects influence interpretation—identical information presented as benefits versus harms elicits different responses.

Conflicting interests among stakeholders create tension. Manufacturers may emphasize benefits while minimizing risks. Patient advocates may demand maximum precaution. Regulators balance protection with access. Effective communication acknowledges these perspectives while prioritizing public health.

Table 18: Elements of Effective Pharmacovigilance Communication

Element	Description	Application
Accuracy	Factually correct, evidence-based content	Verify data sources, cite evidence, acknowledge limitations
Timeliness	Appropriate timing for decision-making	Balance urgency with verification needs
Clarity	Understandable to target audience	Use plain language, define terms, provide examples
Actionability	Clear recommendations for behavior	Specify what recipients should do with information
Context	Adequate background for interpretation	Include comparators, absolute risks, alternatives

10.2 RISK COMMUNICATION STRATEGIES

Risk communication in pharmacovigilance involves conveying information about drug safety concerns to enable informed decision-making while maintaining appropriate medication use and public trust. Effective risk communication requires structured approaches addressing cognitive, emotional, and behavioral dimensions.

Risk Communication Framework

Successful risk communication begins with thorough **risk assessment** establishing what is known about the safety concern, including incidence rates, severity, affected populations, and uncertainties. This evidence base informs subsequent communication.

Message development translates risk assessment into communications appropriate for target audiences. Messages should explain the nature of the risk, who is affected, risk magnitude, comparison with alternatives, risk-benefit balance, and recommended actions.

Channel selection determines how messages reach audiences. Options include direct mailings to healthcare providers, regulatory website postings, professional organization communications, patient information leaflets, media announcements, and social media platforms. Multiple channels ensure broad reach.

Evaluation assesses whether communication achieved objectives through surveys measuring awareness and understanding, monitoring prescribing patterns, tracking adverse event reports, and analyzing media coverage. Evaluation informs future communication improvements.

Framing Risk Information

How risks are presented profoundly influences perception and response. **Absolute risk** expresses event probability in a population (e.g., 1 in 1000 patients). **Relative risk** compares risks between groups (e.g.,

2-fold increase). Both formats provide important information but are interpreted differently.

Natural frequencies (e.g., "1 in 100 patients") are better understood than percentages or probabilities. **Visual representations** including icon arrays or graphs enhance comprehension. **Comparison with familiar risks** provides context, though care is needed selecting appropriate comparators.

Balanced presentation of risks and benefits enables informed decisions. Emphasizing only risks may lead to inappropriate medication discontinuation. Conversely, minimizing risks undermines informed consent.

Addressing Uncertainty

Pharmacovigilance frequently involves uncertain or evolving information. Transparent acknowledgment of uncertainty maintains credibility. Explaining sources of uncertainty (limited data, conflicting studies, biological variability) helps audiences understand limitations.

Avoiding premature definitive statements prevents need for later contradictory communications damaging trust. Conditional language ("current evidence suggests") appropriately conveys uncertainty while providing available information.

Behavioral Recommendations

Effective risk communication includes clear action steps. Vague warnings without guidance create anxiety without enabling appropriate response. Specific recommendations might include continuing medication with increased monitoring, switching to alternative treatments, recognizing warning signs requiring medical attention, or avoiding specific combinations.

Building Trust

Trust forms the foundation for effective risk communication. Consistent, transparent, evidence-based communication builds credibility. Acknowledging mistakes and uncertainties rather than hiding them maintains trust. Independence from commercial interests strengthens credibility. Demonstrating commitment to public welfare over other interests earns confidence.

10.3 COMMUNICATION IN DRUG SAFETY CRISIS MANAGEMENT

Drug safety crises occur when serious, unexpected adverse events emerge, potentially threatening public health and confidence in medication safety. Effective crisis communication minimizes harm while maintaining necessary medication use and public trust in the healthcare system.

Crisis Characteristics

Safety crises typically involve unexpected serious adverse events, high publicity and public concern, uncertainty about risk magnitude and mechanisms, potential for widespread exposure, and need for rapid decision-making with incomplete information. These characteristics demand specialized communication approaches.

Crisis Communication Principles

Rapid response is essential as information vacuums fill with speculation. Initial communications should occur within 24 hours of crisis recognition, even if information is limited. Acknowledging the situation and explaining ongoing investigation maintains credibility.

Consistent messaging across all communicators prevents confusion. Designated spokespersons ensure coordination. Regular updates maintain information flow and demonstrate active management.

Transparency about what is known and unknown builds trust. Hiding information that later emerges destroys credibility far more than initial honesty. Acknowledging uncertainty shows appropriate caution while ongoing investigation continues.

Empathy for affected individuals and concerned stakeholders demonstrates human consideration beyond technical analysis. Acknowledging fears and frustrations while providing reassurance where appropriate balances emotions with facts.

Clear Recommendations

Crisis communications must provide actionable guidance including whether to continue or stop medications, what symptoms warrant medical attention, alternatives for affected patients, and when more information will be available. Ambiguous messages create confusion and inappropriate responses.

Stakeholder Coordination

Effective crisis management requires coordination among regulatory authorities, manufacturers, healthcare professionals, patient groups, and media. Pre-established relationships facilitate rapid coordination during crises. Joint communications prevent contradictory messages.

Post-Crisis Communication

Once immediate crisis passes, follow-up communications provide final risk assessments, lessons learned, system improvements, and appreciation for cooperation. Completing the communication cycle maintains stakeholder relationships for future engagement.

10.4 CRISIS MANAGEMENT PLAN

Structured crisis management plans enable rapid, coordinated responses to drug safety emergencies. Pre-established protocols, roles, and procedures facilitate effective action when time-sensitive decisions are required.

Plan Components

A comprehensive crisis management plan includes crisis definition and categorization, organizational structure and responsibilities, communication protocols and templates, decision-making algorithms, stakeholder contact lists, and evaluation procedures.

Crisis Team

Designated team members with defined roles include a crisis manager coordinating overall response, medical/scientific experts providing technical assessment, regulatory liaison managing authority communication, communications director overseeing messaging, legal counsel ensuring compliance, and senior management providing authorization for major decisions.

Activation Triggers

Clear criteria for plan activation include unexpected serious adverse events, multiple related reports suggesting safety signals, media inquiries about safety concerns, regulatory authority investigations, and public health emergencies involving the product.

Response Protocols

Protocols specify initial assessment procedures, information gathering requirements, internal notification processes, external communication timing, regulatory reporting obligations, and documentation requirements. Templates for communications expedite response while ensuring completeness.

Training and Exercises

Regular training familiarizes team members with plan components. Simulation exercises test plan effectiveness and identify improvements. Scenarios covering various crisis types prepare teams for diverse situations.

10.5 COMMUNICATING WITH REGULATORY AGENCIES

Regulatory authorities require timely, accurate, and complete safety information for oversight responsibilities. Effective communication with regulators combines compliance with reporting requirements and proactive engagement on safety issues.

Regulatory Reporting Requirements

Manufacturers must submit Individual Case Safety Reports (ICSRs) for serious adverse events within specified timeframes—typically 15 days for expedited reports and 90 days for non-expedited reports. Periodic Safety Update Reports (PSURs) or Periodic Benefit-Risk Evaluation Reports (PBRERs) provide comprehensive safety reviews at regular intervals.

Format and Standards

Reports follow standardized formats including ICH E2B for ICSRs and ICH E2C for PSURs. MedDRA terminology ensures consistent coding. Adherence to formatting requirements facilitates regulatory review.

Quality and Completeness

High-quality reports include complete patient information, detailed event descriptions, temporal relationships, dechallenge and rechallenge data, causality assessment, and relevant literature. Incomplete reports delay assessment and may trigger regulatory inquiries.

Proactive Communication

Beyond mandatory reporting, proactive engagement with regulators on emerging signals, planned studies, or risk management strategies demonstrates responsible pharmacovigilance. Early consultation on safety issues facilitates aligned approaches.

Response to Regulatory Inquiries

Timely, thorough responses to regulatory questions demonstrate commitment to safety. Clear explanations of data, limitations, and planned actions address regulatory concerns effectively.

10.6 COMMUNICATION WITH BUSINESS PARTNERS AND STAKEHOLDERS

Pharmaceutical companies collaborate with numerous partners requiring safety information sharing including distributors, contract research organizations, licensors/licensees, and healthcare institutions. Effective communication maintains alignment and ensures appropriate safety management throughout the product lifecycle.

Information Sharing Agreements

Formal agreements specify what safety information will be shared, timelines for communication, responsibilities for reporting, and procedures for managing signals. Clear agreements prevent gaps or duplications in safety monitoring.

Regular Updates

Periodic safety briefings keep partners informed about adverse event trends, ongoing investigations, regulatory communications, and planned risk minimization measures. Shared understanding enables coordinated responses.

Confidentiality and Intellectual Property

Communications must protect confidential business information and proprietary data while ensuring necessary safety information reaches appropriate recipients. Agreements address confidentiality requirements.

10.7 COMMUNICATING WITH HEALTHCARE FACILITIES AND PROFESSIONALS

Healthcare professionals represent critical intermediaries between pharmacovigilance systems and patients. Effective communication with clinicians ensures safety information influences prescribing and monitoring practices.

Educational Communications

Informing healthcare professionals about adverse reactions, risk factors, monitoring recommendations, and management strategies enables optimal medication use. Communications should be evidence-based, practical, and actionable.

Continuing Medical Education

Pharmacovigilance content integrated into continuing education programs reaches professionals regularly. Case-based learning illustrates practical application of safety information.

Clinical Guidelines

Incorporating safety recommendations into treatment guidelines institutionalizes appropriate practices. Collaboration with guideline developers ensures safety evidence informs recommendations.

Feedback Mechanisms

Two-way communication enables healthcare professionals to report observations and ask questions. Responsive engagement builds relationships supporting ongoing safety monitoring.

10.8 MEDIA COMMUNICATION AND PUBLIC AWARENESS

Media serves as the primary channel through which the public learns about drug safety issues. Effective media engagement informs public discourse while preventing misinterpretation and inappropriate alarm.

Media Relations

Designated spokespersons trained in media communication provide consistent messaging. Press releases, press conferences, and interviews deliver information efficiently to media outlets. Preparation for difficult questions enables confident, accurate responses.

Social Media

Digital platforms enable direct public communication but require careful management. Monitoring social media identifies emerging concerns and misinformation. Official social media presence provides authoritative information sources.

Public Awareness Campaigns

Targeted campaigns educate the public about medication safety, adverse event recognition, and reporting systems. Mass media, online platforms, and community outreach reach diverse audiences.

Correcting Misinformation

False or misleading safety information spreads rapidly through social media. Prompt correction with information limits harm. However, debunking misinformation risks amplifying false claims, requiring careful communication strategies.

10.9 DEAR HEALTHCARE PROFESSIONAL COMMUNICATIONS (DHPC)

Dear Healthcare Professional Communications represent formal regulatory-approved letters conveying important drug safety information directly to prescribers. DHPCs address serious safety concerns requiring practice changes.

Purpose and Triggers

DHPCs are issued when significant new safety information emerges that changes the benefit-risk assessment, requires prescribing modifications, identifies previously unrecognized serious risks, or announces major regulatory actions like restrictions or withdrawals.

Development Process

Manufacturers draft DHPCs in consultation with regulatory authorities. Content undergoes regulatory review and approval before distribution. The collaborative process ensures balanced, accurate messaging.

Standard Format

DHPCs follow structured formats including a clear headline summarizing key information, background on the safety concern, summary of new evidence, specific recommendations for practice, and contact information for questions or adverse event reporting.

Distribution Methods

DHPCs reach healthcare professionals through postal mail to licensed prescribers, email to registered healthcare provider lists, professional organization distribution, and posting on regulatory websites. Multiple channels ensure broad reach.

Effectiveness Evaluation

Post-distribution surveys assess whether DHPCs reached intended audiences, were read and understood, and influenced practice. Prescribing pattern analysis determines behavioral impact.

Table 20: DHPC Structure and Content

Section	Content	Purpose
Header	Clear title, product name, date	Immediate identification
Summary Box	Key safety message and recommendations	Quick reference for busy clinicians
Background	Context and previous safety profile	Understanding significance of new information
New Evidence	Data supporting safety concern	Scientific basis for recommendations
Recommendations	Specific practice changes needed	Actionable guidance
Reporting	How to report suspected reactions	Facilitate ongoing surveillance

10.10 RISK MINIMIZATION MEASURES

Risk minimization measures represent systematic interventions reducing adverse event occurrence or severity through targeted communications, educational programs, and restricted access systems. These measures form essential components of comprehensive risk management strategies.

Types of Risk Minimization

Routine measures include approved product information in labeling, package inserts providing comprehensive details, patient information leaflets in lay language, and standard clinical practice guidelines. These measures apply to all medications.

Additional measures address specific serious risks through educational programs for prescribers and patients, restricted distribution systems, pregnancy prevention programs, patient registries, and enhanced monitoring requirements. Regulatory authorities mandate these measures when routine approaches are insufficient.

Educational Materials

Prescriber education includes detailed risk information, patient selection criteria, monitoring recommendations, and management of adverse reactions. Patient education covers risk recognition, importance of monitoring, contraindications, and when to seek medical attention. Validated comprehension testing ensures understanding.

Restricted Access Programs

For medications with serious risks manageable through appropriate use, restricted access ensures only trained prescribers prescribe the drug, patients receive adequate education, and required monitoring occurs. Examples include clozapine registries monitoring for agranulocytosis and isotretinoin pregnancy prevention programs.

Implementation and Monitoring

Effective risk minimization requires systematic implementation including provider enrollment and training, distribution through certified pharmacies, patient enrollment and education, and documentation of compliance. Ongoing evaluation assesses program effectiveness through adverse event monitoring, compliance audits, knowledge assessments, and behavioral surveys.

Modification Based on Outcomes

Risk minimization measures undergo revision based on effectiveness evaluation. Insufficient risk reduction may necessitate more stringent measures. Conversely, if risks prove manageable, requirements may be streamlined.

As pharmacovigilance evolves with expanding data sources, global collaboration, and digital communication channels, communication strategies must adapt while maintaining core principles of accuracy, transparency, and audience-appropriateness. Professionals skilled in pharmacovigilance communication serve vital roles ensuring that safety information achieves its protective purpose - enabling appropriate medication to use that maximizes benefits while minimizing preventable harm.

CHAPTER 11

SAFETY DATA GENERATION

KEY OUTCOMES

Upon completion of this chapter, learners will be able to:

1. Describe the objectives and scope of pre-clinical safety studies
2. Explain various toxicological testing methodologies and their regulatory requirements
3. Understand the role of animal models in predicting human drug safety
4. Differentiate safety monitoring approaches across clinical trial phases
5. Identify safety endpoints and their assessment in clinical research
6. Explain post-marketing surveillance methods and objectives
7. Describe the structure and purpose of PBRERs in ongoing benefit-risk evaluation
8. Understand Development Safety Update Reports in clinical development contexts

ABSTRACT

Safety data generation represents a comprehensive, lifecycle approach to understanding the benefit-risk profile of pharmaceutical products from initial discovery through post-marketing use. This chapter systematically explores the continuum of safety assessment spanning pre-clinical toxicological studies, clinical trial phases, and post-approval surveillance mechanisms. Beginning with animal-based toxicology testing that identifies potential hazards before human exposure, the chapter progresses through the sequential phases of clinical trials where safety is evaluated alongside efficacy in increasingly larger and diverse human populations. Special emphasis is placed on safety endpoints, monitoring strategies, and the critical transition to real-world post-marketing surveillance where rare adverse events and long-term effects emerge. The chapter details regulatory reporting instruments including Periodic Benefit-Risk Evaluation Reports (PBRERs) and Development Safety Update Reports (DSURs) that synthesize accumulating safety data for ongoing risk-benefit assessment, ensuring continuous evaluation throughout a medicine's therapeutic life.

11.1 PRE-CLINICAL PHASE SAFETY STUDIES

Pre-clinical safety studies constitute the essential first step in pharmaceutical development, evaluating drug safety in laboratory and animal models before human exposure. These studies identify potential toxicities, establish safe starting doses for clinical trials, and characterize pharmacokinetic and pharmacodynamic properties.

Objectives and Regulatory Framework

The primary objectives include identifying target organ toxicity, determining dose-response relationships, establishing no-observed-adverse-effect levels (NOAEL), characterizing reversibility of toxic effects, and identifying populations at particular risk. Regulatory authorities including FDA, EMA, and CDSCO require comprehensive pre-clinical safety data before permitting human trials.

Pre-clinical studies follow Good Laboratory Practice (GLP) standards ensuring data quality, integrity, and regulatory acceptability. GLP encompasses organizational structure, personnel qualifications, facility standards, equipment maintenance, standard operating procedures, and documentation requirements.

Study Types and Duration

Pre-clinical safety assessment includes various study types tailored to the intended clinical use. Acute toxicity studies determine effects of single or short-term exposures, typically in two species (rodent and non-rodent), using multiple dose levels to establish lethal dose parameters and identify target organs.

Repeat-dose toxicity studies evaluate effects of repeated exposures over periods ranging from weeks to months. Study duration depends on intended clinical trial duration - short-term studies (2-4 weeks) support Phase I trials of similar duration, while chronic toxicity studies (6-12 months) support long-term clinical development.

Genotoxicity studies assess potential for genetic damage through bacterial mutation tests, chromosomal aberration tests, and in vivo micronucleus tests. These studies identify carcinogenic potential early in development.

Reproductive and developmental toxicity studies evaluate effects on fertility, embryo-fetal development, and pre- and post-natal development. These studies are essential before including women of reproductive potential or pregnant women in clinical trials.

Carcinogenicity studies, required for drugs intended for chronic use, involve long-term (18-24 months) studies in two rodent species to detect tumorigenic potential.

Dose Selection and Extrapolation

Pre-clinical studies typically include a range of doses including the maximum tolerated dose, intermediate doses, and doses producing no observable effects. Human Equivalent Dose (HED) calculations, based on body surface area or allometric scaling, translate animal doses to safe starting doses for human trials, typically incorporating safety factors of 10-fold or greater.

11.2 TOXICOLOGICAL STUDIES

Toxicological studies employ diverse methodologies to comprehensively characterize a drug's potential to cause harm across biological systems and exposure conditions.

General Toxicology

Single-dose toxicity studies identify the dose-response relationship following single administration. Parameters include clinical observations, body weight changes, food consumption, clinical pathology (hematology, clinical chemistry, urinalysis), gross necropsy findings, and organ weights with histopathology.

Repeated-dose toxicity studies assess effects of chronic exposure. Study designs incorporate daily dosing for defined periods (28 days, 90 days, 6 months, or 12 months depending on clinical development plans), with comprehensive monitoring including regular clinical examinations, ophthalmologic examinations, electrocardiography, clinical pathology at intervals, and detailed histopathological evaluation of all tissues.

Genetic Toxicology

Genotoxicity assessment employs a battery of tests addressing different mechanisms of genetic damage. The Ames test detects reverse mutations in bacterial strains. In vitro mammalian cell assays identify chromosomal aberrations or gene mutations. In vivo micronucleus tests detect chromosomal damage in bone marrow or peripheral blood cells of treated animals.

Positive genotoxicity results require further investigation including additional mechanistic studies, dose-response characterization, and potential carcinogenicity assessment.

Reproductive and Developmental Toxicology

Fertility studies assess effects on male and female reproductive function, mating behavior, conception, and early embryonic development. Male fertility studies dose animals before and throughout mating, while female fertility studies dose before mating through implantation.

Embryo-fetal development studies identify potential teratogenic effects through dosing during organogenesis (the period of major organ formation). Pregnant animals receive daily doses during critical developmental windows, with fetuses examined for external, visceral, and skeletal malformations.

Pre- and post-natal development studies evaluate effects on late gestation, parturition, lactation, and offspring development through weaning and maturation. These studies assess maternal toxicity, delivery complications, offspring viability, growth, development, and reproductive capability.

Special Toxicology Studies

Phototoxicity studies evaluate potential for drugs to cause enhanced skin reactions upon light exposure, particularly important for compounds with ultraviolet light absorption characteristics.

Immunotoxicity studies assess effects on immune system function, including immune suppression or enhancement and hypersensitivity potential.

Abuse liability assessment evaluates drugs affecting the central nervous system for dependence potential, involving behavioral studies in animals and subjective effects assessment in early clinical trials.

11.3 ANIMAL MODELS FOR SAFETY ASSESSMENT

Animal models serve as surrogates for predicting human drug responses, though species differences necessitate careful interpretation and extrapolation of findings.

Species Selection

Regulatory guidelines typically require testing in at least two species - one rodent (usually rat or mouse) and one non-rodent (commonly dog or primate). Species selection considers several factors including pharmacological relevance (species with similar drug metabolism and pharmacological response to humans), practical considerations (availability, cost, historical control data), and regulatory requirements.

Rodents offer advantages of relatively low cost, established historical control data, genetic homogeneity in inbred strains, and acceptability for long-term studies including carcinogenicity assessment. However, rodents differ metabolically from humans in important ways.

Non-rodent species such as dogs provide metabolic profiles often more like humans, established pharmacokinetic and toxicological databases, and suitability for cardiovascular and respiratory safety assessment. Non-human primates are used when no other species provides adequate pharmacological relevance, though ethical and practical considerations limit their use.

Limitations and Predictive Value

Animal studies have inherent limitations in predicting human drug responses. Species differences in drug metabolism, pharmacokinetics, target receptor distribution, and disease mechanisms affect translatability. Many human adverse reactions, particularly idiosyncratic reactions, are not detected in animal studies.

Concordance between animal toxicity and human adverse effects varies by reaction type. Target organ toxicity often translates reasonably well, while immunological reactions, idiosyncratic reactions, and psychological effects show poor concordance. Despite limitations, animal studies successfully prevent exposure to severely toxic compounds and identify many clinically relevant safety concerns.

Translational Considerations

Successful translation from animal to human safety requires understanding species-specific factors. Allometric scaling accounts for metabolic rate differences related to body size. Pharmacokinetic modeling helps predict human drug exposure from animal data. Identification of relevant species (those with similar metabolic pathways and pharmacological responses) improves prediction accuracy.

Modern approaches increasingly incorporate in vitro human cell systems, computational modeling, and human tissue-based models (such as organ-on-chip systems) to complement or reduce animal testing while improving human relevance.

11.4 CLINICAL PHASE SAFETY MONITORING

Clinical trials provide the first opportunity to assess drug safety in humans, requiring rigorous monitoring systems to detect, document, and evaluate adverse events while protecting participant welfare.

Ethical and Regulatory Framework

Clinical trial safety monitoring operates within strict ethical and regulatory frameworks. Informed consent ensures participants understand potential risks. Institutional Review Boards (IRBs) or Ethics

Committees review and approve protocols, consent forms, and safety monitoring plans before trial initiation and throughout conduct.

Good Clinical Practice (GCP) guidelines establish international ethical and scientific quality standards for designing, conducting, recording, and reporting clinical trials. GCP ensures participant rights, safety, and **wellbeing take** precedence over scientific interests, and that trial data are credible and accurate.

Safety Monitoring Systems

Effective safety monitoring requires multiple overlapping systems. Routine safety assessments include scheduled visits with targeted questioning, physical examinations, vital signs monitoring, clinical laboratory testing (hematology, chemistry, urinalysis), electrocardiography, and other procedure-specific monitoring based on known drug class effects or pre-clinical findings.

Adverse event collection employs standardized methods including open-ended questioning at each visit, diary completion by participants, and spontaneous reporting encouraged throughout trial participation. Events are documented with details of onset, duration, severity, actions taken, and outcome.

Causality assessment determines the relationship between study drug and adverse events using structured algorithms. Factors considered include temporal relationship, alternative explanations, response to drug discontinuation (dechallenge), response to drug reintroduction (rechallenge if ethically appropriate), known drug effects, and biological plausibility.

Data Safety Monitoring Boards (DSMBs)

For trials with significant risk or long duration, independent Data Safety Monitoring Boards provide ongoing safety oversight. DSMBs comprise experts not involved in trial conduct who periodically review accumulating safety and efficacy data, assess benefit-risk balance, and recommend trial continuation, modification, or termination.

DSMB responsibilities include reviewing serious adverse events, comparing adverse event rates between treatment groups, assessing protocol adherence, and evaluating whether stopping rules (predefined safety or efficacy criteria) have been met.

11.5 PHASE I, II, III, AND IV TRIALS

Clinical development proceeds through sequential phases, each with distinct objectives, populations, and safety monitoring approaches, progressively expanding exposure while gathering evidence for benefit-risk assessment.

Phase I Trials

Phase I trials represent first-in-human studies, typically conducted in 20-100 healthy volunteers (except for cytotoxic drugs tested in patients). Primary objectives include assessing safety and tolerability, characterizing pharmacokinetics, and identifying maximum tolerated dose.

Safety monitoring in Phase I is intensive, often conducted in specialized clinical pharmacology units with continuous medical supervision. Studies employ conservative dose escalation designs starting at fractions of the NOAEL from animal studies. Single ascending dose (SAD) studies evaluate single doses with adequate observation periods before escalating. Multiple ascending dose (MAD) studies assess repeated dosing, monitoring for accumulation and delayed effects.

Phase I trials establish the dose range for later phases but involve limited populations and brief exposure, detecting only acute, common adverse effects. Rare reactions, delayed effects, and reactions in specific populations remain undetected.

Phase II Trials

Phase II trials enroll 100-500 patients with the target condition, focusing on preliminary efficacy assessment while continuing safety evaluation. These trials establish dose-response relationships, optimal dosing regimens, and provide initial benefit-risk assessment in the therapeutic population.

Safety monitoring becomes more comprehensive as exposure duration extends. Phase IIA studies emphasize dose-finding through careful evaluation of efficacy and safety across multiple dose levels. Phase IIB studies evaluate the selected dose(s) in larger patient populations, often including comparators (placebo or active treatment).

Phase II trials detect more adverse effects than Phase I due to longer exposure, larger sample sizes, and inclusion of patients (who may be more vulnerable than healthy volunteers) with concurrent conditions and medications. However, sample sizes remain insufficient for detecting rare reactions

Phase III Trials

Phase III trials represent pivotal studies supporting regulatory approval, enrolling hundreds to thousands of patients in confirmatory efficacy trials that also provide substantial safety databases. These multicenter, often multinational trials closely simulate real-world clinical practice.

Safety monitoring in Phase III emphasizes detecting less common adverse events (occurring in 1 in 100 to 1 in 1000 patients), identifying risk factors for adverse reactions, evaluating long-term safety with extended treatment durations, and assessing safety in diverse populations across age groups, ethnicities, and comorbidities.

Phase III trial designs increasingly incorporate active safety surveillance rather than relying solely on spontaneous reporting. This includes scheduled inquiries about specific adverse events of interest, targeted monitoring based on known class effects or theoretical concerns, and adjudication of selected events by independent experts.

Despite large sample sizes, Phase III trials still cannot detect very rare reactions (less than 1 in 1000), lack adequate representation of some real-world populations, involve selected patients meeting strict eligibility criteria, and have defined treatment durations that may not reflect chronic real-world use.

Phase IV Trials

Phase IV trials or post-marketing studies occur after regulatory approval, addressing questions not fully answered by pre-approval trials. These studies evaluate long-term safety and efficacy, investigate rare adverse events or specific populations, compare different treatment strategies, and assess safety in broader, less selected populations.

Phase IV studies may be voluntary (sponsor-initiated to generate additional evidence) or mandatory (required by regulatory authorities to address specific safety concerns as conditions of approval). Post-authorization safety studies (PASS) specifically address identified or potential risks.

11.6 SAFETY ENDPOINTS IN CLINICAL TRIALS

Safety endpoints define the specific adverse outcomes measured and analyzed in clinical trials, requiring prospective definition in protocols and systematic assessment throughout trials.

Primary Safety Endpoints

Unlike efficacy endpoints where trials typically have one or few primary outcomes, safety assessment involves multiple concurrent endpoints. Adverse event incidence represents the fundamental safety endpoint, documenting all adverse events regardless of causality, serious adverse events specifically, and adverse events leading to treatment discontinuation.

Laboratory parameters serve as objective safety endpoints, with monitoring frequency and specific tests tailored to anticipated drug effects. Clinically significant laboratory abnormalities are predefined (such as liver enzyme elevations exceeding specific thresholds) and require systematic evaluation.

Vital signs and physical findings including blood pressure, heart rate, temperature, weight, and targeted physical examinations provide ongoing safety assessment. Electrocardiographic parameters, particularly QT interval prolongation, receive special attention due to association with dangerous arrhythmias.

Special Safety Endpoints

Certain drugs require endpoint-specific monitoring. Drugs affecting the immune system need detailed immunological assessments. Drugs with abuse potential require systematic evaluation of dependence indicators. Drugs used in pregnancy necessitate pregnancy registries tracking maternal and fetal outcomes.

Suicidality assessment using standardized tools is required for psychiatric drugs and increasingly for other medications with potential central nervous system effects. Malignancy surveillance continues long-term for immunosuppressive agents.

Composite Safety Endpoints

Major adverse cardiovascular events (MACE) represent a composite endpoint commonly used in cardiovascular safety assessment, typically comprising cardiovascular death, myocardial infarction, and stroke. Similar composite endpoints are developed for other organ systems or safety concerns.

11.7 POST-APPROVAL PHASE / POST-MARKETING SURVEILLANCE (PMS)

Post-marketing surveillance represents the critical final phase of safety data generation where medicines are evaluated in real-world clinical practice across broader populations and longer durations than possible in clinical trials.

Rationale and Objectives

Post-marketing surveillance addresses inherent limitations of pre-approval evaluation including detecting rare adverse events not observable in limited trial populations, identifying long-term safety issues requiring years of exposure, evaluating safety in underrepresented populations (children, elderly, pregnant women, patients with multiple comorbidities), assessing safety with concomitant medications and real-world adherence patterns, and detecting safety signals from medication errors, quality defects, or off-label uses.

PMS objectives include continuous benefit-risk monitoring, signal detection and evaluation, risk characterization and quantification, and identification of risk factors and susceptible populations.

Post-Marketing Surveillance Methods

Spontaneous reporting systems constitute the cornerstone of PMS, collecting voluntary reports from healthcare professionals and patients. While cost-effective and capable of detecting rare events, spontaneous reporting suffers from substantial underreporting, incomplete information, and inability to calculate incidence rates without denominator data.

Active surveillance systems proactively collect safety data through various mechanisms. Sentinel systems utilize electronic healthcare databases to monitor defined populations systematically. Registry studies follow patients receiving specific treatments or having specific conditions longitudinally, collecting comprehensive data on outcomes.

Electronic health record (EHR) mining employs computational methods to identify adverse event signals within large healthcare databases. Prescription event monitoring links prescriptions to clinical outcomes in defined populations.

Signal Management in Post-Marketing Phase

Post-marketing signal detection combines quantitative and qualitative approaches. Disproportionality analysis uses statistical methods to identify drug-event combinations reported more frequently than expected. Data mining algorithms screen large databases for potential signals requiring evaluation.

Once signals are detected, systematic signal evaluation determines clinical significance, causality, public health impact, and need for regulatory action. Signal evaluation incorporates literature review, analysis of clinical trial databases, assessment of biological plausibility, and consideration of alternative explanations.

11.8 PERIODIC BENEFIT-RISK EVALUATION REPORTS (PBRER)

The Periodic Benefit-Risk Evaluation Report (PBRER) represents a comprehensive, periodic summary of worldwide safety information for marketed products, facilitating ongoing benefit-risk assessment and regulatory decision-making.

Purpose and Regulatory Framework

PBRERs replaced Periodic Safety Update Reports (PSURs) under ICH E2C(R2) guidelines, representing an evolution toward explicit benefit-risk evaluation rather than mere safety data compilation. Regulatory authorities require PBRERs at defined intervals (typically six-monthly for new products, annually subsequently, with potential for less frequent submission as products mature).

The PBRER serves multiple functions including providing systematic evaluation of product benefit-risk profile, documenting changes in benefit-risk balance since previous reports, communicating new safety information to regulatory authorities, and supporting decisions about product labeling, risk management, or regulatory status.

PBRER Structure and Content

The PBRER follows standardized structure defined in ICH E2C(R2):

Executive Summary provides high-level overview of content, important findings, and conclusions regarding benefit-risk balance.

Introduction establishes context including reporting period dates and covered indications.

Worldwide Marketing Authorization Status documents all countries where the product is approved, approved indications, and significant variations in labeling across regions.

Actions Taken for Safety Reasons describes any regulatory actions, labeling changes, restrictions, or withdrawals during the reporting period.

Changes to Reference Safety Information documents updates to core safety information serving as the reference for expectedness determinations.

Estimated Exposure quantifies patient exposure during the reporting period and cumulatively, typically expressed as patient-years or prescriptions, stratified by indication and region where feasible.

Data Sources describes information sources used including spontaneous reports, clinical trials, literature, and other surveillance activities.

Summary of Significant Findings from Clinical Trials highlights safety findings from ongoing or completed trials during the reporting period.

Findings from Post-Authorization Studies presents results from epidemiological studies, registries, or other post-marketing research.

Other Information includes findings from non-clinical studies, medication error reports, or quality complaints with potential safety implications.

Overall Safety Evaluation provides integrated analysis of all available data, discussing important identified risks, important potential risks, missing information, and any changes in understanding of product safety profile.

Benefit Evaluation separately summarizes evidence for therapeutic benefit including efficacy data, patient-relevant outcomes, and benefit in authorized indications.

Integrated Benefit-Risk Analysis explicitly evaluates whether benefits continue to outweigh risks in authorized indications, considering magnitude of benefit, frequency and severity of risks, availability of therapeutic alternatives, and patient population characteristics.

Conclusions and Actions present overall conclusions about benefit-risk profile and any proposed or planned actions including labeling updates, risk minimization measures, or additional studies.

Signal Evaluation in PBRERs

PBRERs include systematic signal evaluation for new potential safety issues identified during the reporting period. For each signal, the report discusses available evidence, causality assessment, clinical significance, impact on benefit-risk balance, and proposed actions or further investigation needed.

11.9 DEVELOPMENT SAFETY UPDATE REPORT (DSUR)

The Development Safety Update Report (DSUR) serves as the clinical trial equivalent of the PBRER, providing periodic comprehensive safety summaries during drug development.

Purpose and Scope

Established by ICH E2F guidelines, the DSUR harmonizes international requirements for periodic safety reporting during clinical development. The DSUR is submitted annually on the development international birth date (DIBD) - the date of first regulatory approval for clinical trials or the date of first human dosing if no approval is required.

The DSUR aims to provide regulatory authorities with comprehensive annual safety information from all ongoing and completed clinical trials, present cumulative safety data in context, facilitate evaluation of emerging safety profiles, and support decisions about trial continuation or modification.

DSUR Content and Structure

Introduction and Executive Summary provide overview of development status and highlights important safety findings from the reporting period.

Description of Investigational Product and Program includes chemical structure, pharmacological class, formulations, indications under investigation, development phase, and trial status summary.

Marketing Authorization Status documents any marketing approvals obtained during development.

Actions Taken for Safety Reasons describes any regulatory actions, protocol modifications, or clinical holds related to safety.

Changes to Reference Safety Information updates the core safety information used for expectedness determinations in expedited reporting.

Estimated Exposure quantifies subject exposure during the reporting period and cumulatively, typically as subject years stratified by indication and study phase.

Summary of Significant Findings from Clinical Trials presents serious adverse events, other significant adverse events, findings from completed trials, and data from long-term follow-up studies.

Findings from Non-Clinical Studies includes any new toxicology, carcinogenicity, or reproductive toxicity data.

Overall Safety Evaluation provides integrated analysis of accumulating data, discusses emerging safety patterns, evaluates causality for important events, and assesses implications for ongoing and planned trials.

Summary of Important Risks categorizes risks as identified risks (clear evidence from available data), potential risks (suspected but not confirmed), and missing information (gaps in knowledge about specific populations or long-term effects).

Differences Between DSUR and PBRER

While structurally similar, DSURs differ from PBRERs in important ways. DSURs cover investigational products without marketing authorization, focus more heavily on clinical trial data than spontaneous reports, do not include benefit evaluation or formal benefit-risk analysis (since efficacy is not established), and emphasize implications for ongoing development rather than marketed product management.

Safety data emerges across a pharmaceutical product's lifecycle through interconnected phases, each building on the last. Pre-clinical studies in animal models spotlight potential hazards and set safe human trial thresholds, though they can't fully predict our responses. Clinical phases then broaden exposure in diverse groups, mapping safety profiles despite limits in scale, duration, and participant selection. Post-marketing surveillance bridges these gaps, capturing rare events, long-term effects, and issues in real-world, underrepresented populations. Periodic Benefit-Risk Evaluation Reports (PBRERs) for marketed drugs and Development Safety Update Reports (DSURs) for those in trials synthesize this evolving data, enabling ongoing benefit-risk assessments and informed regulatory choices. Together, these vigilant stages - from lab to lifelong use - ensure medicines deliver profound benefits while guarding against preventable harm for all.

CHAPTER 12

ICH GUIDELINES FOR PHARMACOVIGILANCE

KEY OUTCOMES

Upon completion of this chapter, learners will be able to:

1. Explain ICH's organizational structure, membership, and harmonization objectives
2. Describe the ICH harmonization process from concept to guideline implementation
3. Understand expedited reporting requirements for serious adverse events
4. Explain Individual Case Safety Reports structure and regulatory requirements
5. Apply ICH E2A principles for clinical safety data management
6. Describe ICH E2B data elements and electronic transmission standards
7. Understand PSUR/PBRER structure, content, and evaluation principles
8. Apply Good Clinical Practice principles to pharmacovigilance activities

ABSTRACT

The International Council for Harmonisation of Technical Requirements for Pharmaceuticals for Human Use (ICH) has established comprehensive guidelines standardizing pharmacovigilance practices globally. This chapter systematically explores ICH's organizational structure, harmonization processes, and specific pharmacovigilance guidelines that have transformed international drug safety monitoring. Beginning with ICH's formation and objectives, the chapter examines the harmonization process that brings together regulatory authorities and pharmaceutical industry to develop consensus standards. Detailed coverage of individual ICH E2 series guidelines addresses clinical safety data management, electronic transmission standards for individual case safety reports, periodic safety reporting requirements, post-approval safety data management, and pharmacovigilance planning.

12.1 ORGANIZATION AND OBJECTIVES OF ICH

The International Council for Harmonisation (ICH) represents a collaboration between regulatory authorities and pharmaceutical industry aimed at harmonizing technical requirements for drug registration globally. Established in 1990 by regulators from Europe, Japan, and United States along with industry associations, ICH transformed in 2015 into a legal entity with expanded global membership.

Structure and Membership

ICH comprises Regulatory Members (FDA, EMA, PMDA, Health Canada, Swissmedic, MHRA), Industry Members (EFPIA, PhRMA, JPMA), and Observer Organizations (WHO, IFPMA). The Assembly makes policy decisions, the Management Committee oversees operations, and Expert Working Groups develop technical guidelines.

Objectives

ICH aims to harmonize technical requirements for pharmaceutical registration, ensuring safe, effective, and high-quality medicines are developed efficiently. Benefits include reduced duplicate testing, accelerated patient access to new medicines, minimized animal testing, and efficient resource utilization. ICH guidelines, while not legally binding, are adopted into regional regulations, becoming enforceable requirements.

12.2 ICH HARMONIZATION PROCESS

ICH guidelines progress through structured consensus-based stages ensuring scientific validity and regulatory acceptability.

Development Stages

Stage 1 (Concept Paper) identifies need for new guideline with problem description and proposed scope. Stage 2 (Draft Guideline) involves Expert Working Group developing technical content through scientific discussion and consensus building. Stage 3 (Public Consultation) releases draft for stakeholder comment. Stage 4 (Final Guideline) incorporates public comments and achieves regulatory consensus. Stage 5 (Implementation) involves adoption into regional regulations with specified effective dates.

Guideline Categories

ICH organizes guidelines into categories: Quality (Q) addressing pharmaceutical quality, Safety (S) covering non-clinical safety testing, Efficacy (E) addressing clinical trials and pharmacovigilance, and Multidisciplinary (M) covering cross-cutting topics like MedDRA terminology and electronic standards.

12.3 EXPEDITED REPORTING REQUIREMENTS

Expedited reporting ensures rapid communication of serious adverse events from clinical trials and post-marketing use to regulatory authorities and investigators, enabling timely safety assessment and protective actions.

Regulatory Rationale

Expedited reporting serves to alert authorities to potentially serious risks, enable early detection of safety signals, facilitate timely regulatory decisions, and protect trial participants and patients. Rapid reporting is mandated for unexpected serious adverse reactions where speed of communication may influence patient safety.

Criteria for Expedited Reporting

Events requiring expedited reporting must meet specific criteria. In clinical trials, suspected unexpected serious adverse reactions (SUSARs) require expedited reporting - events that are serious, suspected to be drug-related, and unexpected based on reference safety information. In post-marketing, expedited reports are required for serious unexpected adverse reactions occurring during authorized use.

Serious events meet regulatory definitions (death, life-threatening, hospitalization, disability, congenital anomaly, or medically important events). Unexpected events are not described in reference safety information regarding nature, severity, or specificity. Causally related events have reasonable possibility of drug causation based on temporal relationship and lack of alternative explanations.

Reporting Timelines

Regulatory authorities specify maximum reporting timelines. Fatal or life-threatening SUSARs require reporting within 7 calendar days of awareness with complete follow-up within 8 additional days (15-day total). Other serious unexpected adverse reactions require reporting within 15 calendar days of awareness. Follow-up information must be submitted as it becomes available, typically within 15 days of receiving new information.

12.4 INDIVIDUAL CASE SAFETY REPORTS (ICSRs)

Individual Case Safety Reports provide standardized documentation of single suspected adverse drug reactions, enabling systematic collection, transmission, and analysis of safety information globally.

ICSR Components

A complete ICSR contains four essential elements: identifiable patient (age, sex, initials or identifier), identifiable reporter (healthcare professional or consumer), suspected drug(s) with administration details, and adverse event(s) with description and outcome.

Additional information enhances assessment value including medical history, concomitant medications, event chronology with dates, laboratory/diagnostic findings, causality assessment, seriousness and expectedness determinations, and outcome with recovery status.

ICSR Lifecycle

ICSRs progress through defined stages. Initial report contains minimum required elements submitted within regulatory timelines. Follow-up reports provide additional information obtained after initial submission, with significant new information requiring expedited follow-up. Final report documents complete case information including outcome and causality conclusion.

12.5 ICH E2A: CLINICAL SAFETY DATA MANAGEMENT

ICH E2A establishes definitions and standards for clinical safety data management during drug development, providing foundation for harmonized safety assessment and reporting.

Key Definitions

ICH E2A standardizes critical terminology. Adverse Event (AE) is any untoward medical occurrence in a patient administered a pharmaceutical product, not necessarily causally related. Adverse Drug Reaction (ADR) is a response to a drug that is noxious and unintended, occurring at normal doses. Unexpected Adverse Reaction has nature or severity inconsistent with reference safety information. Serious Adverse Event/Reaction meets specific regulatory criteria for severity.

Safety Data Collection and Documentation

E2A recommends systematic adverse event collection through non-leading questions at each patient contact, standardized documentation forms, consistent terminology and coding using MedDRA, and complete information including onset, duration, severity, action taken, and outcome. Clinical trials should specify which adverse events are solicited versus spontaneously reported, define monitoring frequency and methods, and establish clear causality assessment procedures.

Reporting Responsibilities

Sponsor responsibilities include establishing pharmacovigilance systems, ensuring timely regulatory reporting, notifying investigators and ethics committees, maintaining safety databases, and conducting ongoing benefit-risk evaluation. Investigator responsibilities include reporting all serious adverse events immediately to sponsor, documenting all adverse events on case report forms, following up events to resolution, and assessing causality.

12.6 ICH E2B: DATA ELEMENTS FOR TRANSMISSION OF ICSR

ICH E2B specifies standardized data elements for electronic transmission of Individual Case Safety Reports, enabling automated exchange between sponsors and regulatory authorities worldwide.

E2B Structure

E2B defines comprehensive data elements organized in hierarchical structure including administrative information, patient demographics, reaction/event information, drug/medication information, narrative description, sender and receiver information, and medical history/concurrent conditions.

Each data element has specified format (text, date, coded term), size limitations, mandatory or optional status, and repeatability. The standard uses Message Specification for Electronic Transmission enabling computer-to-computer exchange in standardized format (E2B(R2) uses ICH format; E2B(R3) uses ISO/HL7 standard).

Implementation Benefits

E2B implementation enables automated report receipt and processing, reduces data entry errors, facilitates international data exchange, enables efficient database searches, and supports statistical signal detection. Most regulatory authorities require E2B-formatted submissions, with E2B(R3) increasingly mandated globally.

12.7 ICH E2C: PSURs/PBRERs

ICH E2C(R2) establishes standards for periodic safety reporting of marketed medicines through Periodic Benefit-Risk Evaluation Reports (PBRERs), evolution from earlier Periodic Safety Update Reports.

PSUR to PBRER Evolution

Original PSURs focused primarily on safety data compilation. E2C(R2) transformed this to PBRERs emphasizing explicit benefit-risk evaluation, integration of benefit and risk data, structured signal evaluation, and harmonized submission frequencies.

Core Principles

PBRERs provide comprehensive review of benefit-risk profile at regular intervals, highlight changes since previous report, present integrated benefit-risk analysis, and document actions taken or planned. Reports should be concise, analytical rather than descriptive, focused on clinically relevant findings, and supported by appropriate data.

Table 21: PBRER Reporting Cycle

Product Age	Reporting Frequency	Rationale
First 2 years post-approval	Every 6 months	New products require intensive monitoring
Next 2 years (years 3-4)	Annually	Moderate monitoring as safety profile clarifies
After 4 years	Every 3 years	Established products with stable profiles

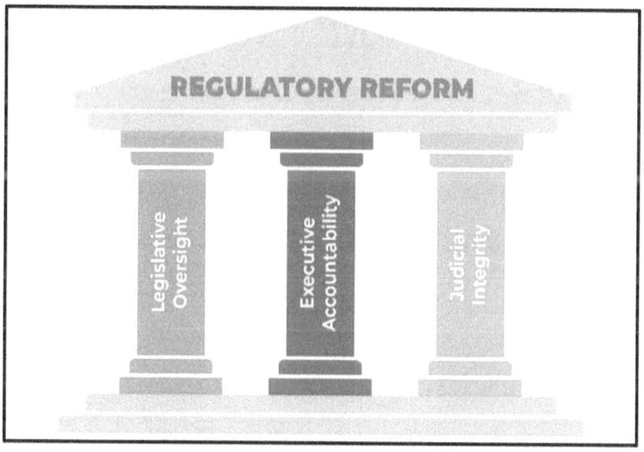

Figure 13: PBRER submission frequency decreases as products mature and safety profiles become well-characterized. Regulatory authorities may modify frequencies based on safety concerns.

12.8 PSUR/PBRER STRUCTURE AND CONTENT

Major PBRER Sections

Executive Summary provides concise overview of important findings and benefit-risk conclusions. Worldwide Marketing Authorization Status documents all approved countries, indications, and significant regional variations. Actions Taken for Safety Reasons describes regulatory actions, labeling changes, or restrictions during reporting period.

Estimated Exposure quantifies patient exposure using prescription data, sales data, or patient registries, expressed as patient-years or treatment episodes. Summary of Clinical Trials highlights safety findings from ongoing and completed trials. Post-Authorization Safety Studies presents results from epidemiological studies and registries.

Overall Safety Evaluation integrates all safety data discussing important identified risks, important potential risks, and missing information. Benefit Evaluation summarizes evidence for therapeutic efficacy. Integrated Benefit-Risk Analysis explicitly evaluates whether benefits continue to outweigh risks in approved indications.

12.9 POST-APPROVAL EXPEDITED REPORTING

Post-approval expedited reporting requirements ensure rapid communication of serious safety information from marketed products to regulatory authorities.

Reporting Criteria

Serious unexpected adverse reactions from any source (spontaneous reports, literature, post-authorization studies) require expedited reporting. Events must be serious, unexpected relative to approved labeling, and have reasonable causal relationship to the product. Companies must establish systems to identify reportable cases among all received adverse event reports.

Timelines and Formats

Fatal and life-threatening unexpected reactions require initial report within 15 days for most authorities. Other serious unexpected reactions require reporting within 15 days. Reports follow ICSR format per E2B specifications. Follow-up information must be submitted promptly as it becomes available.

12.10 ICH E2D: POST-APPROVAL SAFETY DATA MANAGEMENT

ICH E2D addresses definitions and standards for post-approval safety data management, complementing E2A which focuses on pre-approval clinical development.

Key Concepts

E2D emphasizes that safety monitoring continues throughout product lifecycle. Post-approval data sources include spontaneous reports, literature, post-authorization studies, and reports from health authorities.

Companies must maintain pharmacovigilance systems capable of receiving, processing, evaluating, and reporting safety information from all sources globally.

Data Handling Requirements

Organizations must establish processes for case triage (determining reportability), follow-up (obtaining additional information), evaluation (causality and seriousness assessment), and timely reporting to authorities. Duplicate reports must be identified and consolidated. Quality assurance procedures ensure data accuracy and completeness.

12.11 ICH E2E: PHARMACOVIGILANCE PLANNING

ICH E2E provides guidance on planning pharmacovigilance activities throughout product development and post-approval, integrating safety considerations into overall development strategy.

Pharmacovigilance Planning Principles

Effective pharmacovigilance requires prospective planning, not reactive responses. Planning should begin in early development, be updated as knowledge evolves, integrate pre-clinical and clinical data, address identified and potential risks, and specify risk minimization measures.

Safety Specification

The Safety Specification identifies important identified risks (clear evidence of causation), important potential risks (concern but not confirmed), and missing information (gaps in knowledge about special populations or long-term effects). This specification guides surveillance priorities and risk management planning.

12.12 RISK MANAGEMENT PLAN (RMP)

Risk Management Plans provide comprehensive frameworks for identifying, characterizing, preventing, and managing medication risks throughout product lifecycle.

RMP Structure

Module I: Safety Specification documents important risks and missing information. Module II: Pharmacovigilance Plan describes activities for monitoring and further characterizing risks including routine pharmacovigilance, additional monitoring activities, and post-authorization safety studies. Module III: Risk Minimization Measures describes interventions to prevent or reduce risk occurrence or severity including routine measures (labeling, pack size restrictions) and additional measures (controlled distribution, pregnancy prevention programs, patient registries).

RMP Development and Updates

RMPs are initially submitted with marketing authorization applications and updated when new safety information emerges, risk minimization measures are modified, results from pharmacovigilance activities become available, or at regulatory milestones. RMPs represent living documents evolving with accumulating knowledge.

Table 22: Risk Management Plan Components

Module	Component	Purpose
I	Safety Specification	Identifies known risks, potential risks, missing information
II	Pharmacovigilance Plan	Describes routine and additional monitoring activities

III	Risk Minimization	Details measures to prevent or reduce risks
--	Effectiveness Evaluation	Assesses whether risk minimization achieves objectives

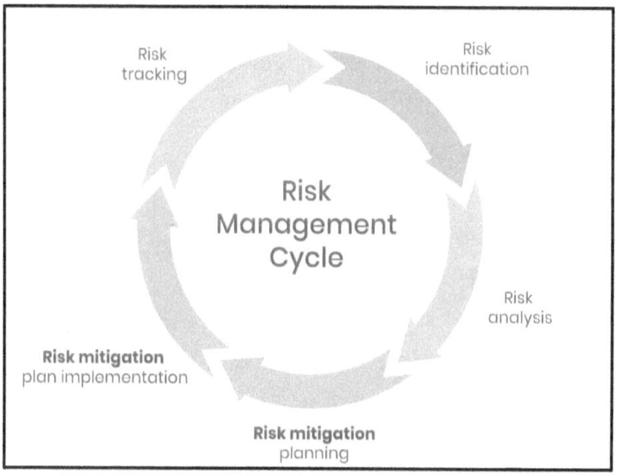

Figure 14: The RMP integrates risk identification, monitoring, and mitigation in systematic framework, with continuous evaluation ensuring interventions achieve intended safety objectives.

12.13 GOOD CLINICAL PRACTICE (GCP) IN PHARMACOVIGILANCE STUDIES

Good Clinical Practice principles apply not only to efficacy trials but also to pharmacovigilance studies including post-authorization safety studies, pregnancy registries, and active surveillance programs.

GCP Principles

Clinical trials and pharmacovigilance studies must protect participant rights, safety, and wellbeing; be scientifically sound with clear objectives; be conducted by qualified personnel; obtain ethical review and informed consent; maintain data quality and integrity; and comply with regulatory requirements. These principles ensure that safety data are reliable and ethically obtained.

Application to Pharmacovigilance

Post-authorization safety studies require protocol development specifying objectives, design, and methods; ethics committee approval; informed consent when directly contacting patients; data quality assurance; and reporting of serious adverse events. Registry studies need clear protocols, participant consent procedures, standardized data collection, and periodic evaluation of findings.

12.14 ICH E6: GOOD CLINICAL PRACTICE GUIDELINES

ICH E6 establishes international ethical and scientific quality standards for designing, conducting, recording, and reporting clinical trials involving human subjects.

Fundamental Principles

Trials should be scientifically justified, described in clear protocol, approved by ethics committee, conducted by qualified investigators, with voluntary informed consent from participants. Participant wellbeing takes precedence over science and society interests. Data must be accurate, complete, and verifiable.

Responsibilities

Sponsors ensure qualified investigators, provide adequate resources, establish data management systems, monitor trial conduct, and ensure regulatory compliance. Investigators protect participant safety, obtain informed consent, report adverse events, maintain accurate records, and follow protocol. Ethics Committees review protocols, consent processes, and trial conduct to protect participants.

Documentation Requirements

Essential documents including protocol, informed consent forms, investigator qualifications, ethics approvals, case report forms, adverse event reports, monitoring logs, and final reports must be maintained. Documentation enables reconstruction of trial conduct and verification of data integrity.

ICH guidelines have fundamentally transformed global pharmacovigilance through harmonized standards that facilitate international collaboration, reduce duplicate efforts, and enhance drug safety monitoring. The E2 series guidelines establish comprehensive frameworks spanning clinical development through post-marketing surveillance, addressing expedited reporting, standardized case documentation, periodic safety reporting, and pharmacovigilance planning. Implementation of these guidelines ensures consistent safety assessment across regions while allowing regulatory flexibility for local requirements.

Good Clinical Practice principles embedded within ICH guidelines ensure that safety data are generated ethically and meet quality standards essential for regulatory decision-making. As pharmacovigilance continues evolving with technological advances and expanding data sources, ICH guidelines provide stable yet adaptable frameworks supporting the fundamental objective of protecting public health through systematic medication safety monitoring. Understanding and applying these harmonized standards is essential for pharmacovigilance professionals working in increasingly globalized pharmaceutical development and regulatory environments.

CHAPTER 13

PHARMACOGENOMICS OF ADVERSE DRUG REACTIONS

KEY OUTCOMES

Upon completion of this chapter, learners will be able to:

1. Explain fundamental concepts of pharmacogenomics and their relevance to ADRs
2. Describe how genetic variations influence drug response and adverse reactions
3. Identify major cytochrome P450 polymorphisms affecting drug metabolism
4. Understand HLA typing applications in predicting immune-mediated ADRs
5. Recognize biomarkers for ADR susceptibility in clinical practice
6. Apply pharmacogenomic principles toward personalized medicine and ADR prevention

ABSTRACT

Pharmacogenomics represents the convergence of pharmacology and genomics, exploring how genetic variations influence individual responses to medications, including susceptibility to adverse drug reactions. This chapter examines the fundamental principles of pharmacogenomics and its application in predicting, preventing, and managing ADRs. Beginning with genetic variations affecting drug metabolism and response, the chapter explores cytochrome P450 polymorphisms, pharmacokinetic and pharmacodynamic variations, and the role of HLA typing in predicting severe immune-mediated reactions. The integration of biomarkers for ADR susceptibility and the evolution toward personalized medicine demonstrate how genetic information can optimize therapeutic outcomes while minimizing adverse events. Understanding pharmacogenomic principles enables healthcare professionals to implement precision medicine approaches, tailoring drug selection and dosing to individual genetic profiles for enhanced safety and efficacy.

13.1 INTRODUCTION TO PHARMACOGENOMICS

Pharmacogenomics is the study of how genes affect a person's response to drugs, combining pharmacology and genomics to develop effective, safe medications and doses tailored to individual genetic makeup. While traditional pharmacology assumes relatively uniform drug responses across populations, clinical experience reveals substantial inter-individual variability in both therapeutic efficacy and adverse effects.

Genetic factors account for 20-95% of variability in drug disposition and effects, depending on the specific medication. This genetic influence operates through multiple mechanisms including variations in drug-metabolizing enzymes, drug transporters, drug targets (receptors), and immune response genes. Pharmacogenomics seeks to identify these genetic determinants and translate them into clinical tools for optimizing drug therapy.

The field distinguishes between pharmacogenetics (studying single gene effects on drug response) and pharmacogenomics (examining multiple genes and genome-wide influences). However, these terms are often used interchangeably in clinical contexts. The goal is implementing personalized or precision medicine, where therapeutic decisions incorporate individual genetic information alongside clinical factors.

Historical milestones include recognition of genetic influences on drug metabolism in the 1950s, identification of specific polymorphisms in the 1970s-1980s, completion of the Human Genome Project in 2003 providing comprehensive genetic maps, and subsequent integration of pharmacogenomic testing into clinical guidelines for numerous medications.

13.2 GENETIC VARIATIONS AND ADRs

Genetic variations occur throughout the human genome, with several types particularly relevant to drug response and ADR susceptibility. Single nucleotide polymorphisms (SNPs) represent the most common genetic variations, where a single DNA base differs among individuals. While most SNPs have no functional consequences, those occurring in genes encoding drug-metabolizing enzymes, transporters, or targets can significantly affect drug response.

Copy number variations (CNVs) involve deletions or duplications of gene segments, potentially resulting in absent, reduced, normal, or increased gene expression. For drug-metabolizing enzymes, CNVs can create poor metabolizers (no functional copies) or ultra-rapid metabolizers (multiple gene copies).

Insertions and deletions (indels) add or remove DNA segments, potentially disrupting gene function. Other variations include microsatellite repeats, chromosomal rearrangements, and epigenetic modifications affecting gene expression without altering DNA sequence.

These genetic variations influence ADR risk through multiple pathways. Altered drug metabolism resulting from enzyme polymorphisms can cause drug accumulation (poor metabolizers) increasing toxicity risk, or rapid drug clearance (ultra-rapid metabolizers) reducing efficacy. Modified drug transport affects tissue distribution and elimination. Changed drug target sensitivity alters therapeutic and adverse response intensity. Immune system variations, particularly in human leukocyte antigen (HLA) genes, influence susceptibility to immune-mediated ADRs.

Population differences in allele frequencies mean certain genetic variants are more common in specific ethnic groups, contributing to observed population-based differences in ADR rates. For instance, HLA-B*1502 associated with carbamazepine-induced Stevens-Johnson syndrome is prevalent in Asian populations but rare in Europeans.

13.3 GENETICS-RELATED ADRs WITH EXAMPLES

Numerous well-characterized genetic associations with ADRs demonstrate pharmacogenomics' clinical relevance. Abacavir hypersensitivity provides a paradigm example - this antiretroviral drug causes severe hypersensitivity reactions in approximately 5-8% of patients, strongly associated with the HLA-B*5701 allele. Pre-treatment screening and avoiding abacavir in positive patients virtually eliminates this reaction, representing pharmacogenomics' success in ADR prevention.

Carbamazepine-induced severe cutaneous reactions including Stevens-Johnson syndrome and toxic epidermal necrolysis show strong association with HLA-B*1502 in Han Chinese and Southeast Asian populations. Regulatory agencies recommend HLA-B*1502 screening before initiating carbamazepine in at-risk populations.

Warfarin-related bleeding risk relates to polymorphisms in CYP2C9 (metabolizing enzyme) and VKORC1 (warfarin target). Patients with reduced-function CYP2C9 variants or certain VKORC1 variants require lower doses to avoid excessive anticoagulation and bleeding. FDA-approved warfarin labeling includes dosing tables incorporating genetic information.

Thiopurine toxicity (used in leukemia and inflammatory bowel disease) correlates with TPMT (thiopurine methyltransferase) polymorphisms. Poor metabolizers accumulate toxic metabolites causing severe myelosuppression. TPMT testing guides dose adjustment, preventing life-threatening hematological toxicity.

Simvastatin myopathy risk increases with SLCO1B1 polymorphisms affecting drug uptake into hepatocytes, leading to higher systemic exposure and muscle toxicity. Genetic testing identifies patients requiring alternative statins or lower doses.

Clopidogrel treatment failure relates to CYP2C19 polymorphisms. Clopidogrel requires CYP2C19-mediated activation; poor metabolizers have reduced active metabolite formation, inadequate platelet inhibition, and increased cardiovascular event risk. Alternative antiplatelet agents may be preferred in poor metabolizers.

13.4 PHARMACOKINETIC (PK) PARAMETERS AND GENETIC POLYMORPHISM

Pharmacokinetics describes drug absorption, distribution, metabolism, and excretion - all influenced by genetic polymorphisms affecting relevant proteins. Absorption variations relate to transporter polymorphisms affecting intestinal uptake. For example, P-glycoprotein (encoded by ABCB1) transports numerous drugs; genetic variants alter expression and function, affecting oral bioavailability.

Distribution depends on plasma protein binding and tissue transporters. Polymorphisms in genes encoding albumin, alpha-1-acid glycoprotein, or tissue transporters modify drug distribution, affecting free (active) drug concentrations and tissue exposure.

Metabolism represents the most extensively studied pharmacogenomic area. Phase I metabolism (primarily oxidation via cytochrome P450 enzymes) and Phase II metabolism (conjugation reactions) exhibit substantial genetic variability. Polymorphisms create metabolizer phenotypes ranging from poor to ultra-rapid, dramatically affecting drug clearance and systemic exposure.

Excretion involves renal and biliary transporters with genetic variants influencing drug elimination rates. Organic anion transporters (OATs), organic cation transporters (OCTs), and efflux transporters show polymorphisms affecting renal and hepatic drug clearance.

These pharmacokinetic variations manifest clinically as altered drug exposure. Poor metabolizers experience higher drug concentrations from standard doses, increasing ADR risk. Conversely, ultra-rapid metabolizers may have subtherapeutic concentrations, risking treatment failure. Genetic testing combined with therapeutic drug monitoring optimizes dosing for individuals with variant phenotypes.

13.5 CYP450 ENZYME POLYMORPHISMS

Cytochrome P450 (CYP450) enzymes constitute the major drug-metabolizing system, responsible for metabolizing approximately 75% of clinically used drugs. These enzymes, primarily hepatic but present in other tissues, catalyze oxidation reactions converting lipophilic drugs to more water-soluble metabolites for elimination.

The CYP450 superfamily includes numerous isoforms, with CYP1A2, CYP2C9, CYP2C19, CYP2D6, and CYP3A4/5 accounting for most drug metabolism. Each enzyme exhibits genetic polymorphisms creating metabolizer phenotypes with clinical significance.

CYP2D6 represents the most polymorphic drug-metabolizing enzyme, with over 100 identified allelic variants. Despite metabolizing only 20-25% of drugs, CYP2D6 substrates include important cardiovascular drugs (beta-blockers, antiarrhythmics), antidepressants, antipsychotics, and opioids. Approximately 7-10% of Caucasians are CYP2D6 poor metabolizers (PM), experiencing increased adverse effects from standard doses. Conversely, ultra-rapid metabolizers (carrying gene duplications) may require higher doses for therapeutic effect but risk toxicity from prodrugs requiring CYP2D6 activation (e.g., codeine converted to morphine).

CYP2C9 metabolizes drugs including warfarin, phenytoin, NSAIDs, and oral hypoglycemics. The CYP2C9*2 and *3 variants have reduced enzymatic activity. Patients with reduced-function alleles require lower warfarin doses to avoid bleeding, lower phenytoin doses to prevent neurotoxicity, and potentially experience increased NSAID-related GI bleeding.

CYP2C19 metabolizes proton pump inhibitors, clopidogrel, certain antidepressants, and benzodiazepines. Poor metabolizers (15-20% of Asians, 2-5% of Caucasians) have impaired clopidogrel activation, reduced antiplatelet effect, and increased cardiovascular event risk. Conversely, poor metabolizers respond better to PPIs due to reduced drug clearance.

CYP3A4/5 metabolize approximately 50% of drugs but show less clinically significant polymorphism than other CYPs, though activity varies considerably due to genetic and environmental factors including drug interactions and induction.

Clinical implementation includes genotype-guided dosing for drugs with significant CYP450-mediated metabolism, particularly those with narrow therapeutic indices or where standard dosing causes frequent ADRs. Pharmacogenomic consortia provide evidence-based guidelines for genotype-informed prescribing.

13.6 PHARMACODYNAMIC VARIATIONS

While pharmacokinetic variations affect drug concentrations, pharmacodynamic variations alter drug effects at given concentrations by modifying drug targets, downstream signaling pathways, or physiological response mechanisms. Polymorphisms in genes encoding drug receptors, ion channels, enzymes targeted by drugs, or signaling molecules influence therapeutic and adverse responses.

Receptor polymorphisms include beta-adrenergic receptor variants affecting cardiovascular drug responses, opioid receptor variants influencing analgesic efficacy and adverse effects, and dopamine receptor variants modifying antipsychotic response and side effect profiles.

Ion channel polymorphisms, particularly in cardiac potassium channels (HERG/KCNH2), influence susceptibility to drug-induced QT prolongation and potentially fatal arrhythmias. Patients with congenital long QT syndrome variants show heightened sensitivity to QT-prolonging drugs.

Target enzyme polymorphisms include VKORC1 variants affecting warfarin sensitivity, ACE variants influencing ACE inhibitor response, and methylenetetrahydrofolate reductase (MTHFR) variants affecting methotrexate toxicity and folate requirements.

These pharmacodynamic variations often show ethnic differences, contributing to population-based response variations. Integration with pharmacokinetic information provides comprehensive understanding of individual drug response profiles.

13.7 HLA TYPING AND ADR PREDICTION

Human leukocyte antigen (HLA) genes encode major histocompatibility complex (MHC) proteins presenting antigens to T cells, initiating immune responses. HLA molecules are highly polymorphic, with different alleles influencing immune recognition patterns. Specific HLA alleles strongly associate with severe immune-mediated ADRs, enabling prediction and prevention through pre-treatment screening.

The mechanism involves drug or drug-metabolite binding to specific HLA molecules, altering their structure or peptide-binding properties. This creates new antigens recognized by T cells, triggering immune responses manifesting as hypersensitivity, severe cutaneous reactions, or organ-specific toxicity.

Established HLA-ADR associations include HLA-B*5701 and abacavir hypersensitivity (nearly 100% sensitivity), HLA-B*1502 and carbamazepine-induced Stevens-Johnson syndrome/toxic epidermal necrolysis in Asian populations, HLA-B*5801 and allopurinol-induced severe cutaneous reactions, and HLA-A*3101 and carbamazepine hypersensitivity in European populations.

Clinical implementation requires HLA typing before initiating specific drugs in at-risk populations. Regulatory labels recommend or mandate screening for certain drug-HLA combinations. Positive patients should avoid the associated drug, as no safe dose exists - these reactions are not dose-dependent.

13.8 BIOMARKERS FOR ADR SUSCEPTIBILITY

Biomarkers are measurable indicators of biological states or conditions, used in pharmacovigilance to predict, detect, or monitor ADRs. Genetic biomarkers discussed previously represent one category; others include biochemical, molecular, or physiological markers indicating ADR risk or occurrence.

Predictive biomarkers identify patients at higher ADR risk before drug initiation, including genetic markers (CYP450 genotypes, HLA alleles), baseline biochemical values (liver enzymes, renal function), and patient characteristics (age, comorbidities). These enable preventive strategies through patient selection, dose adjustment, or enhanced monitoring.

Diagnostic biomarkers detect ADRs early, often before clinical manifestation, including liver enzyme elevations indicating hepatotoxicity, cardiac troponins suggesting cardiotoxicity, and inflammatory markers signaling immune-mediated reactions.

Monitoring biomarkers track ADR progression or resolution, including drug concentrations (therapeutic drug monitoring), organ function tests, and specific toxicity markers.

Implementation challenges include validation requirements, cost-effectiveness considerations, accessibility of testing, and integration into clinical workflows. Despite challenges, biomarker-guided approaches increasingly enable personalized ADR prevention and management strategies.

13.9 PERSONALIZED MEDICINE AND ADR PREVENTION

Personalized medicine (also termed precision medicine) tailors' medical treatment to individual patient characteristics, incorporating genetic information, biomarkers, clinical factors, and environmental influences. In pharmacovigilance, personalized approaches aim to optimize drug safety by identifying high-risk individuals before ADR occurrence and adjusting treatment accordingly.

Implementation strategies include pre-emptive pharmacogenomic testing, where genetic variants affecting multiple drugs are identified before prescribing, enabling genotype-guided decisions across therapeutic areas throughout patient lifetime. Reactive testing performs genetic analysis when ADRs occur, guiding alternative therapy selection and informing future prescribing. Phenotype-based approaches use clinical characteristics, disease biomarkers, and prior drug responses to guide therapy without genetic testing.

Current applications with strong evidence include thiopurine dosing based on TPMT genotype, anticoagulation guided by CYP2C9/VKORC1 variants, HLA screening before abacavir or carbamazepine, and CYP2C19-guided antiplatelet therapy selection. Clinical decision support systems increasingly incorporate pharmacogenomic information, providing point-of-care guidance.

Barriers to widespread implementation include testing costs, limited awareness among prescribers, lack of standardized interpretation, reimbursement issues, and ethical considerations regarding genetic information. Ongoing research expands the evidence base, guidelines provide implementation frameworks, and technology facilitates integration into routine practice.

The future envisions routine genetic profiling informing drug selection and dosing throughout healthcare, substantially reducing ADR burden through anticipatory, individualized therapeutic strategies.

Pharmacogenomics has transformed understanding of ADR causation, revealing genetic underpinnings of inter-individual variability in drug response. From cytochrome P450 polymorphisms affecting metabolism to HLA variants predicting immune-mediated reactions, genetic factors substantially influence ADR susceptibility. Clinical implementation through pre-treatment screening, genotype-guided dosing, and biomarker monitoring enables personalized approaches preventing many serious ADRs. As evidence expands, costs decrease, and integration improves, pharmacogenomic-guided therapy will increasingly become standard practice, fulfilling personalized medicine's promise of maximizing therapeutic benefit while minimizing adverse effects for each individual patient.

CHAPTER 14

DRUG SAFETY EVALUATION IN SPECIAL POPULATIONS

KEY OUTCOMES

Upon completion of this chapter, learners will be able to:

1. Describe age-related pharmacokinetic differences affecting drug safety in pediatric patients
2. Understand challenges and safety implications of off-label drug use in children
3. Explain FDA pregnancy categories and current pregnancy-lactation labeling approaches
4. Identify teratogenic drugs and principles of drug safety during pregnancy
5. Assess drug safety during breastfeeding and factors affecting infant exposure
6. Describe physiological changes in elderly patients affecting drug disposition
7. Recognize polypharmacy risks and drug interaction patterns in geriatric populations
8. Apply specialized pharmacovigilance approaches for vulnerable populations

ABSTRACT

Special populations including pediatric patients, pregnant and lactating women, and elderly individuals present unique challenges in drug safety evaluation due to physiological differences affecting pharmacokinetics and pharmacodynamics, limited clinical trial representation, and heightened vulnerability to adverse drug reactions. This chapter systematically examines drug safety considerations across these populations, exploring age-related pharmacokinetic variations in children, off-label medication uses in pediatrics, teratogenic risks during pregnancy, drug transfer in lactation, and the complex interplay of physiological aging, polypharmacy, and increased ADR susceptibility in geriatric patients. Understanding population-specific factors enables appropriate drug selection, dosing adjustments, enhanced monitoring, and informed risk-benefit assessments, ensuring optimal therapeutic outcomes while minimizing preventable harm in vulnerable patient groups requiring specialized pharmacovigilance approaches.

A. PEDIATRICS

Pediatric patients, ranging from premature neonates through adolescents, represent a heterogeneous population with developmental stage-specific physiological characteristics affecting drug disposition, response, and adverse reaction patterns. Children are not simply "small adults" - significant pharmacokinetic and pharmacodynamic differences necessitate specialized approaches to drug therapy and safety monitoring.

14.1 AGE-RELATED PHARMACOKINETIC DIFFERENCES

Pediatric pharmacokinetics differ substantially from adults, varying across developmental stages from neonatal period through adolescence. These differences affect all pharmacokinetic parameters—absorption, distribution, metabolism, and excretion.

Absorption variations in neonates and infants include higher gastric pH (approaching adult values by 2-3 years), affecting ionization and solubility of drugs; prolonged gastric emptying time increasing absorption variability; irregular peristalsis affecting intestinal transit; and immature intestinal enzyme systems modifying pre-systemic metabolism. These factors cause unpredictable oral bioavailability for many drugs. Intramuscular absorption may be erratic due to limited muscle mass and variable perfusion. Percutaneous absorption is enhanced in neonates due to thinner, more hydrated skin with greater surface area relative to body weight, increasing systemic exposure and toxicity risk from topically applied medications.

Distribution differences reflect altered body composition throughout development. Neonates have higher total body water (70-75% vs. 50-60% in adults) requiring larger initial doses of hydrophilic drugs to achieve therapeutic concentrations. Fat content is lower in neonates (10-15%) than adults (20-30%), affecting distribution of lipophilic drugs. Plasma protein binding is reduced due to lower albumin concentrations, different protein characteristics, and competing bilirubin binding, resulting in higher free drug fractions and increased pharmacological effects or toxicity risk. The blood-brain barrier is more permeable in neonates, allowing greater CNS drug penetration and neurotoxicity susceptibility.

Metabolism undergoes significant maturation. Phase I reactions (CYP450 enzymes) show reduced activity in neonates, with different isoforms maturing at varying rates - CYP3A7 (fetal form) predominates initially, gradually replaced by CYP3A4 through infancy; CYP2D6 reaches adult capacity by 3-5 years; CYP2E1 matures by 1 year. This immaturity prolongs drug half-lives, necessitating dose reductions or interval extensions. Phase II conjugation reactions (glucuronidation, sulfation) also mature postnatally, with glucuronidation particularly immature in neonates (explaining chloramphenicol toxicity - "gray baby syndrome"). Some metabolic pathways transiently exceed adult capacity during childhood, requiring higher weight-adjusted doses of certain medications.

Excretion maturation affects renal drug elimination. Glomerular filtration rate is approximately 30-40% of adult values at birth, reaching adult levels (adjusted for body surface area) by 6-12 months. Tubular secretion and reabsorption mature more slowly. Reduced renal function necessitates dose adjustments for renally eliminated drugs in neonates and young infants, with careful monitoring to avoid accumulation and toxicity.

14.2 PEDIATRIC ADR REPORTING

Pediatric patients experience unique adverse drug reaction patterns reflecting developmental pharmacology, off-label medication use, and specific vulnerabilities. However, pediatric ADRs remain underreported compared to adult populations, limiting safety knowledge.

Pediatric-specific ADRs include gray baby syndrome from chloramphenicol (impaired glucuronidation), Reye's syndrome associated with aspirin use during viral infections, tetracycline-induced teeth discoloration and bone growth inhibition, fluoroquinolone-related cartilage toxicity, and increased sensitivity to opioid-induced respiratory depression. Growth and development complications represent pediatric-specific concerns - corticosteroids affecting linear growth, antiepileptic drugs impacting cognitive development, and chemotherapy causing long-term effects on organ development and function.

Reporting challenges include recognition difficulties (children may not verbalize symptoms), attribution complexity (symptoms may be attributed to underlying disease), limited caregiver awareness of reporting systems, and hesitancy among healthcare providers to report suspected reactions in children. Off label use further complicates ADR assessment, as reactions may be "expected" in labeled populations but unexpected when drugs are used outside approved indications or age groups.

Enhancing pediatric pharmacovigilance requires increased healthcare provider education about pediatric-specific ADRs, simplified reporting mechanisms accessible to parents and caregivers, active surveillance in pediatric settings, and mandatory pediatric development plans requiring post-marketing surveillance in children. Regulatory initiatives in various countries incentivize pediatric drug studies, gradually expanding labeled pediatric indications and improving safety knowledge.

14.3 OFF-LABEL USE IN CHILDREN

Off-label drug use refers to prescribing medications for indications, age groups, doses, or durations not included in approved product labeling. Off-label use is particularly prevalent in pediatrics, with estimates suggesting 50-70% of medications administered to hospitalized children and higher proportions in neonatal intensive care units are used off-label.

Reasons for off-label use include limited pediatric clinical trial participation historically (due to ethical concerns, recruitment challenges, and lack of commercial incentives), many conditions affecting children lacking approved pediatric treatments, and developmental differences requiring dose modifications not reflected in labeling.

Safety implications are significant. Off-label medications lack pediatric-specific dosing information, increasing dosing error risk. Safety data in children are limited, and adverse effects may differ from adult patterns. Efficacy may not translate from adults to children due to developmental differences in disease pathophysiology and drug response.

Risk mitigation strategies include basing off label prescribing on published evidence, clinical experience, or expert recommendations; using standardized dosing resources (pediatric formularies, dosing calculators); implementing enhanced monitoring for efficacy and adverse effects; engaging in shared decision-making with parents/caregivers, discussing limited safety data; and reporting observed ADRs to contribute to safety knowledge. Regulatory reforms in the US (Best Pharmaceuticals for Children Act, Pediatric Research Equity Act) and Europe (Pediatric Regulation) have increased pediatric drug development, gradually reducing off-label use necessity for common conditions.

B. PREGNANCY AND LACTATION

Pregnancy and lactation present unique drug safety considerations. Maternal-fetal-infant unit involves complex pharmacokinetic changes, developing fetal vulnerability, and infant exposure through breast milk. Balancing maternal therapeutic needs against potential fetal or infant harm requires careful risk-benefit assessment.

14.4 FDA PREGNANCY CATEGORIES (HISTORICAL)

The US FDA historically used pregnancy categories (A, B, C, D, X) from 1979 to 2015 to communicate fetal risk. Though replaced by narrative labeling, understanding these categories remains relevant as they appear in older literature and clinical decision tools.

Category A: Adequate, well-controlled studies in pregnant women showed no risk to the fetus. Very few drugs achieved this classification due to ethical challenges conducting controlled studies in pregnant women.

Category B: Animal studies showed no fetal risk, but human studies are lacking, OR animal studies showed risk but well-controlled human studies did not confirm risk. Most used category, though providing limited guidance.

Category C: Animal studies showed adverse fetal effects, but human studies are lacking, OR no animal or human studies exist. Risk cannot be ruled out, but potential benefits may justify use. Largest category, offering minimal decision-making guidance.

Category D: Positive evidence of human fetal risk exists, but potential benefits may warrant use in serious conditions lacking safer alternatives (e.g., certain antiepileptics, chemotherapy).

Category X: Studies in animals or humans demonstrated fetal abnormalities, or evidence of fetal risk exists, and risks clearly outweigh any possible benefits. Contraindicated in pregnancy (e.g., thalidomide, isotretinoin).

Limitations included oversimplification of complex risk-benefit analyses, lack of risk severity gradation within categories, no distinction between indication severity, and missing information about critical exposure windows. These limitations led to category system replacement.

In 2015, FDA implemented the Pregnancy and Lactation Labeling Rule (PLLR), replacing categories with narrative sections: pregnancy (including labor and delivery), lactation, and females and males of reproductive potential. This approach provides comprehensive, evidence-based information about risks, dosing considerations, and data quality, enabling informed clinical decisions.

14.5 TERATOGENICITY AND EMBRYOTOXICITY

Teratogenicity refers to drug-induced structural or functional abnormalities in the developing embryo or fetus. Embryotoxicity encompasses broader adverse effects including growth restriction, functional impairment, or fetal death. Susceptibility varies dramatically based on gestational timing.

Critical periods include pre-implantation (conception to ~2 weeks): "all-or-none" period where exposure either causes embryonic death or no effect due to pluripotent cell compensation. Embryonic period (weeks 3-8): organogenesis occurs; maximum sensitivity to structural malformations as organs form. Specific organs are vulnerable during their formation periods. Fetal period (weeks 9 to term): structural malformations are less likely; functional deficits, growth restriction, and minor morphological abnormalities may occur.

Known teratogenic drugs include thalidomide (limb defects, organ malformations), isotretinoin (craniofacial, cardiac, thymic abnormalities), valproic acid (neural tube defects, developmental delays), warfarin (skeletal and CNS abnormalities - "fetal warfarin syndrome"), ACE inhibitors (renal dysgenesis, oligohydramnios when exposed in second/third trimesters), and certain antineoplastic agents causing multiple malformations.

Risk assessment principles include avoiding teratogenic drugs during pregnancy when possible, using alternative safer medications, limiting use to situations where benefits clearly outweigh risks with informed consent, employing lowest effective doses for shortest durations, and timing treatment outside critical developmental windows when feasible.

Prevention strategies involve pre-conception counseling for women of childbearing potential using teratogenic medications, reliable contraception while taking teratogenic drugs, pregnancy testing before initiating high-risk medications, and risk management programs for drugs like isotretinoin (iPLEDGE program).

14.6 DRUG SAFETY DURING BREASTFEEDING

Most drugs transfer into breast milk to some degree, potentially exposing nursing infants. However, actual infant exposure depends on multiple factors, and most medications are compatible with breastfeeding with appropriate precautions.

Factors affecting milk transfer include maternal factors (dose, frequency, pharmacokinetics), drug properties (molecular weight - smaller molecules transfer more readily; lipid solubility - lipophilic drugs enter milk more easily; protein binding - highly bound drugs transfer less; ionization - weak bases concentrate in milk which is slightly acidic), and timing (peak maternal plasma concentrations correspond to highest milk levels).

Infant exposure assessment considers relative infant dose (RID) - ratio of infant's dose via milk to maternal dose, both weight-adjusted. Generally, RID < 10% is considered acceptable. Absolute infant dose depends on milk consumption volume (~150 mL/kg/day). Infant's ability to metabolize and eliminate the drug affects systemic exposure and toxicity risk - neonates with immature metabolism face higher risks than older infants.

Drugs contraindicated or requiring caution include cytotoxic chemotherapy, certain psychotropic medications (lithium), amiodarone, some sedatives/hypnotics causing infant sedation, drugs of abuse, and radioactive compounds. Most common medications (antibiotics, analgesics, antihypertensives) are compatible with breastfeeding, particularly when used short-term.

Risk minimization involves selecting drugs with shorter half-lives, lower oral bioavailability (less infant absorption even if present in milk), and preferably with established breastfeeding safety data. Timing feeds to avoid peak drug levels (taking medication immediately after feeding), monitoring infant for effects (sedation, feeding changes, rashes), and considering temporary pumping and discarding milk during short-term medication courses allows medication use while protecting infant safety.

C. GERIATRICS

Elderly patients (typically defined as ≥65 years) represent the fastest-growing population segment and the highest medication users yet face disproportionate ADR burden. Age-related physiological changes, multiple comorbidities, and polypharmacy create complex pharmacological challenges.

14.7 AGE-RELATED PHYSIOLOGICAL CHANGES

Aging affects all organ systems, with substantial inter-individual variability. Pharmacokinetic and pharmacodynamic changes increase ADR susceptibility.

Pharmacokinetic changes include altered absorption (decreased gastric acid production, reduced splanchnic blood flow, slowed GI motility - generally minor impact on extent of absorption though rate may decrease), distribution modifications (decreased lean body mass and total body water reducing distribution volume of hydrophilic drugs, increased body fat increasing distribution volume of lipophilic drugs with prolonged half-lives, reduced serum albumin increasing free fractions of acidic drugs), metabolic decline (hepatic mass and blood flow decrease, Phase I metabolism (CYP450) capacity declines variably while Phase II metabolism is relatively preserved - metabolism-dependent drugs show prolonged half-lives), and reduced excretion (renal function declines progressively - glomerular filtration, tubular secretion, and reabsorption decrease; creatinine clearance may decline 30-50% by age 80, though serum creatinine may remain normal due to reduced muscle mass; renally eliminated drugs accumulate, requiring dose adjustments).

Pharmacodynamic changes alter drug sensitivity independent of pharmacokinetics. Increased CNS sensitivity to sedatives, opioids, and anticholinergics increases cognitive impairment and fall risk. Altered cardiovascular reflexes impair compensation for orthostatic hypotension caused by antihypertensives or psychotropics. Changed receptor numbers or function affect drug response. Reduced homeostatic reserve limits physiological compensation when drugs cause perturbations.

14.8 POLYPHARMACY AND DRUG INTERACTIONS

Polypharmacy, typically defined as concurrent use of five or more medications, is prevalent in elderly patients with multiple chronic conditions. While often clinically indicated, polypharmacy substantially increases ADR and drug interaction risks.

Consequences include increased ADR incidence (risk rises exponentially with medication number), drug-drug interactions (pharmacokinetic interactions altering drug concentrations, pharmacodynamic interactions causing additive or antagonistic effects), prescribing cascades (ADRs misattributed to new conditions, prompting additional medications), medication errors (complex regimens reducing adherence, increasing administration errors), and functional decline (cumulative drug effects causing cognitive impairment, falls, frailty).

High-risk medications in elderly include anticholinergic drugs (cognitive impairment, constipation, urinary retention), benzodiazepines (falls, fractures, cognitive decline), antipsychotics (increased mortality, stroke risk, falls), NSAIDs (GI bleeding, renal impairment, cardiovascular events), and first-generation antihistamines (sedation, anticholinergic effects).

The Beers Criteria and STOPP/START criteria identify potentially inappropriate medications in elderly populations, guiding deprescribing and safer alternatives. Regular medication review, discontinuing unnecessary drugs, simplifying regimens, and prioritizing drugs with best benefit-risk profiles reduce polypharmacy harms.

14.9 ADRs IN ELDERLY POPULATIONS

Elderly patients experience 2-3 times higher ADR incidence than younger adults, with serious reactions more common and outcomes more severe.

Common ADRs include falls and fractures (from sedatives, antihypertensives, psychotropics), delirium and cognitive impairment (anticholinergics, benzodiazepines, opioids), GIbleeding (NSAIDs, anticoagulants, antiplatelets), renal impairment (NSAIDs, ACE inhibitors, diuretics), electrolyte disturbances (diuretics, lithium), and orthostatic hypotension (antihypertensives, antipsychotics, antidepressants).

Risk factors beyond age include multiple medications, comorbidities, cognitive impairment affecting medication management, living alone with limited supervision, previous ADR history, renal or hepatic impairment, and frailty. Female gender shows higher ADR rates, possibly due to pharmacokinetic differences, higher medication use, or reporting patterns.

Prevention strategies require comprehensive geriatric assessment before initiating medications, "start low, go slow" dosing approach beginning with lower doses and titrating gradually, regular medication review with deprescribing unnecessary drugs, avoiding high-risk medications when safer alternatives exist, monitoring renal function and adjusting doses accordingly, patient and caregiver education about ADR recognition and reporting, and simplifying regimens to enhance adherence and reduce errors.

Special considerations include recognizing atypical ADR presentations in elderly patients - nonspecific symptoms like confusion, weakness, or functional decline may represent drug toxicity rather than disease progression. Drug-disease interactions where medications worsen existing conditions (anticholinergics in dementia, NSAIDs in heart failure) require vigilance. Transitions of care represent high-risk periods for medication errors and ADRs, necessitating medication reconciliation.

Enhanced monitoring in geriatric patients includes baseline and periodic assessment of renal and hepatic function, regular review of indication continuation (is drug still needed?), monitoring for drug accumulation with renally cleared medications, screening for cognitive changes and functional decline, and active ADR surveillance with lower thresholds for suspecting drug involvement in new symptoms.

Special populations - pediatric, pregnant and lactating women, and elderly patients - present unique pharmacovigilance challenges requiring specialized knowledge and approaches. Developmental differences in children, from neonatal through adolescent periods, dramatically affect drug disposition and response, necessitating age-appropriate dosing, heightened ADR surveillance, and cautious off-label use with enhanced safety monitoring. Pregnancy involves complex risk-benefit assessments balancing maternal therapeutic needs against potential teratogenic or embryotoxic effects, guided by gestational timing and exposure circumstances. Breastfeeding safety evaluation requires understanding drug transfer into milk and infant exposure assessment, though most medications are compatible with nursing when appropriately selected and used.

Elderly patients face compounded risks from age-related physiological changes affecting pharmacokinetics and pharmacodynamics, multiple comorbidities requiring multiple medications (polypharmacy), and reduced physiological reserve limiting tolerance for adverse effects. These populations historically were underrepresented in clinical trials, creating knowledge gaps that pharmacovigilance must address through enhanced post-marketing surveillance, specialized reporting systems, and population-specific research.

Optimal care requires recognizing population-specific vulnerabilities, applying appropriate dosing adjustments based on developmental stage or age-related changes, selecting medications with best safety profiles when alternatives exist, implementing enhanced monitoring strategies, and maintaining vigilance for atypical ADR presentations. Healthcare providers must balance therapeutic necessity against potential harms, engage in shared decision-making with patients or caregivers, and contribute to pharmacovigilance systems through diligent ADR reporting. As populations age globally and neonatal survival improves, special population pharmacovigilance will increasingly influence public health outcomes, making specialized knowledge essential for all healthcare professionals involved in medication therapy management.

Special populations - children, pregnant and lactating women, and the elderly - demand tailored pharmacovigilance, as their unique biology reshapes drug behavior and risks. In pediatrics, from fragile neonates to growing adolescents, developmental shifts in drug handling call for precise dosing, vigilant ADR watch, and careful off-label use. Pregnancy weighs maternal needs against fetal threats like teratogenicity, timed by gestational stage, while breastfeeding scrutinizes milk transfer to safeguard infants - most drugs prove safe with wise choices.

The elderly grapple with physiologic decline, polypharmacy amid comorbidities, and frail reserves that amplify ADR impact. Long underrepresented in trials, these groups rely on post-marketing surveillance, targeted reporting, and dedicated research to close knowledge gaps.

Safeguarding them means spotting vulnerabilities, tweaking doses for age or stage, prioritizing safer options, ramping up monitoring, and decoding unusual ADRs. Providers must weigh benefits against harms, partner in decisions with patients or caregivers, and fuel pharmacovigilance via reporting. As global aging accelerates and more neonates thrive, mastering this domain becomes every clinician's imperative for better outcomes.

Table 23: Pharmacokinetic Changes Across Age Groups

Parameter	**Pediatric (Neonates/Infants)**	**Adults**	**Geriatric (≥65 years)**
Body water	Increased (70-75%)	Normal (50-60%)	Decreased (45-55%)
Body fat	Decreased (10-15%)	Normal (20-30%)	Increased (25-40%)
Protein binding	Decreased	Normal	Decreased
Hepatic metabolism	Immature, variable	Mature	Reduced Phase I
Renal function	Immature (matures by 1 year)	Normal	Progressively declines

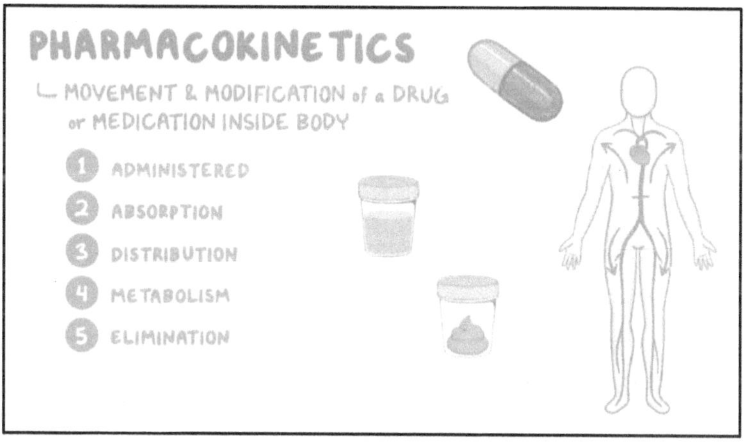

Figure 15: This comparison illustrates how pharmacokinetic parameters vary systematically across age groups, explaining differential drug disposition and ADR susceptibility in vulnerable populations.

Table 24: Critical Periods of Teratogenic Susceptibility During Pregnancy

Gestational Period	Timeframe	Teratogenic Susceptibility	Examples of Vulnerable Organs
Pre-implantation	0-2 weeks	All-or-none effect	Embryo survival vs. loss
Embryonic (Organogenesis)	3-8 weeks	Maximum structural defects	Heart (weeks 3-7), CNS (weeks 3-6), limbs (weeks 4-8), palate (weeks 6-8)
Fetal	9 weeks to term	Functional defects, growth	CNS function, reproductive organs

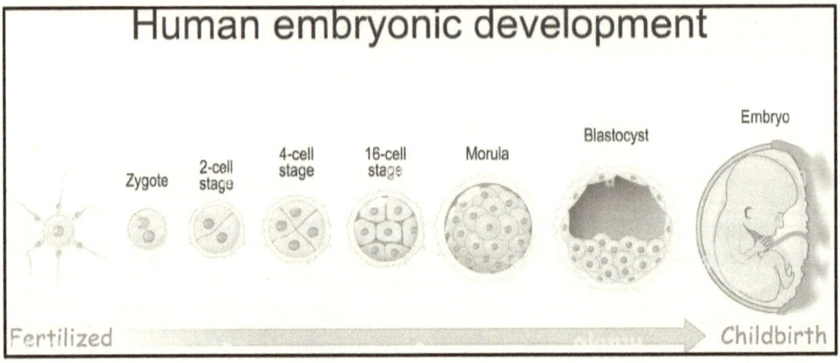

Figure 16: Teratogenic susceptibility varies dramatically throughout gestation, with the embryonic period representing maximum vulnerability to structural malformations during organogenesis.

Table 25: Factors Contributing to Increased ADR Risk in Elderly Patients

Factor Category	Specific Contributors	Clinical Impact
Physiological	Reduced renal clearance, decreased hepatic metabolism, altered body composition	Increased drug concentrations, prolonged half-lives
Multiple medications	Polypharmacy, complex regimens	Drug interactions, medication errors, non-adherence
Comorbidities	Multiple chronic conditions, organ impairments	Altered drug response, drug-disease interactions
Frailty	Reduced homeostatic reserve, cognitive decline	Decreased tolerance, impaired compensation, poor outcomes

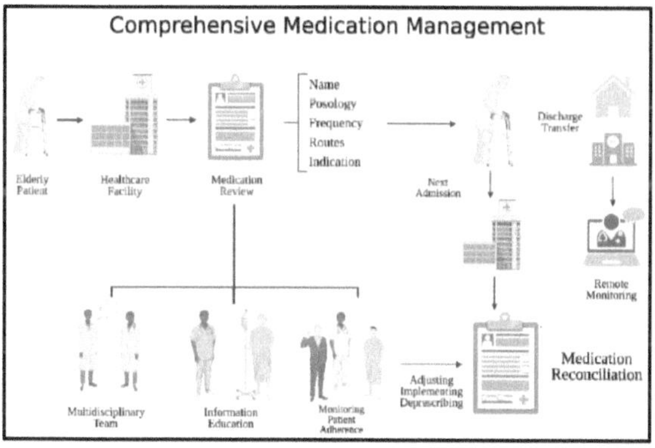

Figure 17: Multiple interconnected factors create a cumulative vulnerability to adverse drug reactions in elderly populations.

CHAPTER 15

CIOMS (COUNCIL FOR INTERNATIONAL ORGANIZATIONS OF MEDICAL SCIENCES

KEY OUTCOMES

Upon completion of this chapter, learners will be able to:

1. Understand CIOMS role in international pharmacovigilance harmonization
2. Describe CIOMS Working Groups and their contributions
3. Explain key recommendations from CIOMS reports I-XII
4. Apply the CIOMS I Form for ADR reporting
5. Prepare Core Clinical Safety Information (CCSI)
6. Implement signal detection and evaluation principles
7. Conduct benefit-risk assessments

ABSTRACT

The Council for International Organizations of Medical Sciences (CIOMS) is a pivotal international body that harmonizes pharmacovigilance practices globally. Established in 1949 under WHO and UNESCO, CIOMS develops practical guidelines through expert working groups. This chapter covers CIOMS Working Groups, the evolution of CIOMS reports I-XII, the standardized CIOMS Form for ADR reporting, guidelines for Core Clinical Safety Information, and methodologies for signal detection and benefit-risk assessment. These CIOMS contributions form the backbone of international drug safety harmonization and regulatory alignment.

15.1 INTRODUCTION TO CIOMS

The Council for International Organizations of Medical Sciences (CIOMS) is an international non-governmental organization founded in 1949 under WHO and UNESCO. CIOMS facilitates collaboration between regulatory authorities, pharmaceutical industry, and healthcare professionals to harmonize pharmacovigilance practices globally.

CIOMS addresses practical challenges in drug safety through expert consensus, develops standardized reporting formats, and bridges regulatory differences across countries. The organization operates through specialized Working Groups that produce comprehensive reports on specific pharmacovigilance topics. These reports have become foundational references for regulatory agencies worldwide, including FDA, EMA, and CDSCO.

15.2 CIOMS WORKING GROUPS

CIOMS Working Groups comprise international experts from regulatory agencies, pharmaceutical companies, academia, and healthcare institutions. Each group focuses on specific pharmacovigilance topics and develops practical guidance through consensus-building.

Working groups typically include 15-25 members representing diverse geographical regions and professional backgrounds. They meet regularly over 2-4 years to review scientific literature, analyze current practices, and develop recommendations. The collaborative nature ensures that guidance reflects both regulatory requirements and practical feasibility.

Recent working groups have addressed topics including individual case safety reports, periodic safety update reports, signal detection methodologies, vaccine safety, pharmacogenomics, benefit-risk assessment, drug-drug interactions, and safety in special populations.

15.3 CIOMS I TO CIOMS XII REPORTS

CIOMS has published twelve major reports addressing evolving pharmacovigilance challenges:

CIOMS I (1990): Introduced the standardized CIOMS Form for international exchange of individual case safety reports. This single-page format revolutionized adverse event reporting and remains widely used for expedited reporting.

CIOMS II (1992): Addressed periodic safety update reports, establishing the foundation for modern PSURs. Recommended standardized formats for summarizing post-marketing safety data at regular intervals.

CIOMS III (1995): Focused on guidelines for preparing Core Clinical Safety Information (CCSI) and Core Data Sheets, standardizing how safety information is presented globally.

CIOMS IV (1998): Examined benefit-risk assessment methodologies, providing frameworks for systematic evaluation of medicinal product value.

CIOMS V (2001): Addressed current challenges in pharmacovigilance, including signal detection, data quality, and international collaboration issues.

CIOMS VI (2005): Focused on management of safety information from clinical trials, establishing principles for unblinding, reporting, and safety data handling during development.

CIOMS VII (2006): Examined Development Safety Update Reports (DSURs), standardizing safety reporting during clinical development phases.

CIOMS VIII (2010): Addressed practical aspects of signal detection in pharmacovigilance, providing methodologies for identifying and evaluating potential safety issues.

CIOMS IX (2012): Focused on practical approaches to risk minimization for medicinal products, including risk management planning and evaluation.

CIOMS X (2016): Examined evidence synthesis and meta-analysis for drug safety, providing guidance on systematic reviews and quantitative evidence integration.

CIOMS XI (2019): Addressed patient involvement in drug development and pharmacovigilance, recognizing the growing importance of patient-reported outcomes and patient engagement.

CIOMS XII (2022): Focused on benefit-risk balance for medicinal products in the real-world setting, emphasizing post-authorization safety assessment and evidence generation.

15.4 CIOMS FORM FOR ADR REPORTING

The CIOMS Form is a standardized one-page reporting format designed for international exchange of suspected adverse drug reaction reports. Introduced in CIOMS I report, it facilitates rapid communication of serious adverse events between countries and organizations.

The form captures essential information including patient demographics (age, sex, weight), suspected adverse reaction details (description, onset date, outcome), suspected and concomitant medications (dose, route, dates), relevant medical history, reporter information, and manufacturer details.

The CIOMS Form is particularly valuable for expedited reporting of serious adverse events between pharmaceutical companies and regulatory authorities. It provides a concise summary while ensuring all critical data elements are communicated. The form has been adapted by many organizations while maintaining its core structure.

15.5 CIOMS I FORM STRUCTURE

The CIOMS I Form follows a logical structure divided into distinct sections:

Section 1 - Patient Information: Includes patient initials, age/date of birth, sex, weight, and height. Protects patient confidentiality while providing demographic data essential for safety assessment.

Section 2 - Adverse Reaction: Describes the reaction(s), onset date, severity, outcome (recovered, recovering, not recovered, fatal, unknown), and whether the event was serious according to regulatory criteria.

Section 3 - Suspected Drug(s): Lists suspected medicinal products with dose, route, frequency, indication for use, therapy dates, and actions taken (drug withdrawn, dose reduced, dose increased, dose not changed, unknown).

Section 4 - Concomitant Medication: Documents other drugs taken by the patient, including dose, route, indication, and therapy dates.

Section 5 - Medical History: Relevant medical conditions, allergies, and previous adverse reactions.

Section 6 - Additional Information: Includes rechallenge information, laboratory data, autopsy findings, and narrative description of the event.

Section 7 - Reporter Information: Reporter's name, address, profession, and report date.

Section 8 - Manufacturer Information: Manufacturer receipt date, report type (initial/follow-up), case reference number, and sender details.

Table 26: CIOMS I Form Key Sections

Section	Content	Purpose
Patient Information	Demographics, initials	Identify patient characteristics
Adverse Reaction	Event description, outcome, seriousness	Document the adverse event
Suspected Drug(s)	Product details, dosing, therapy dates	Identify causative medication
Concomitant Medication	Other drugs taken	Assess drug interactions
Medical History	Pre-existing conditions	Evaluate alternative causes
Additional Information	Lab data, rechallenge, narrative	Provide clinical context

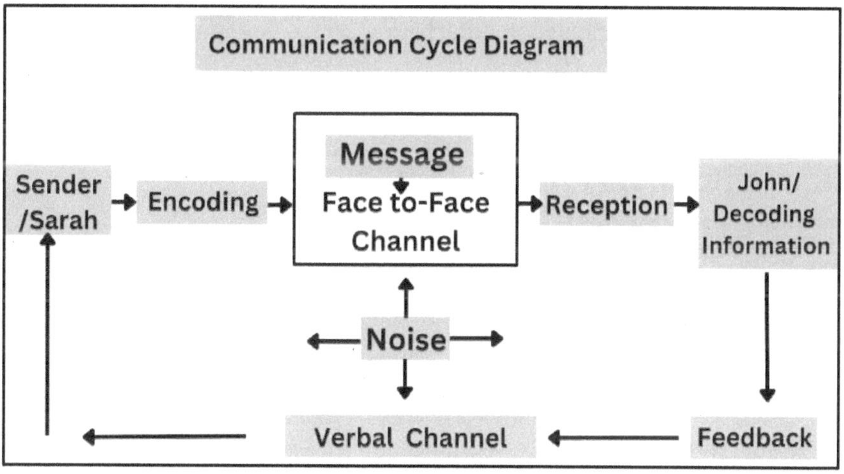

Figure 18: This table outlines the essential sections of the CIOMS I Form, demonstrating how each component contributes to comprehensive adverse event documentation while maintaining a concise one-page format suitable for rapid international exchange.

15.6 GUIDELINES FOR PREPARING CORE CLINICAL SAFETY INFORMATION

Core Clinical Safety Information (CCSI) is a comprehensive compilation of safety data derived from clinical trials and post-marketing experience, presented in standardized format. CIOMS III report established principles for preparing CCSI.

CCSI serves as the reference safety information for a medicinal product globally and forms the basis for Company Core Data Sheets (CCDS). The CCSI includes contraindications, warnings and precautions, adverse reactions organized by frequency and severity, special populations considerations (pregnancy, lactation, pediatrics, geriatrics), and overdose management information.

Preparation requires systematic review of all available safety data from clinical trials, spontaneous reports, literature, and other sources. Information is categorized by organ system using standardized terminology (MedDRA). Adverse reaction frequencies are classified as very common (≥1/10), common (≥1/100 to <1/10), uncommon (≥1/1000 to <1/100), rare (≥1/10,000 to <1/1000), and very rare (<1/10,000).

CCSI must be updated regularly to reflect new safety information. CIOMS recommends annual review or more frequently when significant new safety data emerges.

15.7 SIGNAL DETECTION AND EVALUATION

Signal detection is the process of identifying new, potentially causal associations between drugs and adverse events. CIOMS VIII report provided comprehensive guidance on practical signal detection methodologies.

A signal is defined as information arising from one or multiple sources suggesting a new potentially causal association between a drug and adverse event that is judged to be of sufficient likelihood to justify verification.

Signal Detection Methods:

Spontaneous reporting analysis involves reviewing individual case safety reports for unusual patterns, serious outcomes, or unexpected events. Qualitative review by experienced safety professionals remains fundamental.

Statistical methods include disproportionality analysis using measures like Proportional Reporting Ratio (PRR), Reporting Odds Ratio (ROR), and Bayesian methods (IC, EBGM). These quantify whether an adverse event is reported more frequently than expected for a particular drug.

Data mining techniques systematically screen large databases to identify drug-event combinations warranting further evaluation. Algorithms compare observed versus expected reporting frequencies.

Signal Evaluation Process:

Once detected, signals undergo systematic evaluation: data validation confirms case quality and causality, additional data sources are reviewed (literature, clinical trials), clinical assessment evaluates biological plausibility and temporal relationships, epidemiological evaluation determines true incidence rates, and regulatory impact assessment decides if action is needed.

Signal prioritization considers severity of the event, preventability, population exposure, strength of evidence, regulatory history, and public health impact.

15.8 BENEFIT-RISK ASSESSMENT

Benefit-risk assessment systematically evaluates whether a medicinal product's therapeutic benefits outweigh its potential harms. CIOMS IV and XII reports provided frameworks for conducting benefit-risk evaluations throughout product lifecycle.

Key Components:

Benefit identification includes therapeutic effects (efficacy in treating disease), symptom relief, improved quality of life, prevention of disease progression, and reduced mortality or morbidity.

Risk identification encompasses adverse drug reactions (frequency, severity, reversibility), drug interactions, contraindications in vulnerable populations, potential for abuse or dependence, and long-term safety concerns.

Benefit-Risk Balance is not static but evolves with:

- Additional clinical experience and post-marketing data
- Identification of new risks or benefits
- Changes in available therapeutic alternatives
- Evolving disease understanding
- Shifts in population exposure patterns

Structured Frameworks:

CIOMS recommends structured approaches including defining decision context, identifying relevant benefits and risks, measuring and estimating effects, integrating evidence, and communicating findings transparently.

Quantitative methods may include multi-criteria decision analysis, which weights different benefit and risk outcomes according to their importance. Visual representations like forest plots, effect tables, and benefit-risk maps aid communication.

Benefit-risk assessment informs regulatory decisions at marketing authorization, label updates, risk management measures, and market withdrawal when risks exceed benefits.

CIOMS has fundamentally shaped modern pharmacovigilance through systematic development of practical, consensus-based guidelines. The CIOMS reports provide internationally recognized frameworks for adverse event reporting, periodic safety assessments, signal detection, and benefit-risk evaluation. The CIOMS I Form remains a cornerstone of international safety reporting, enabling rapid exchange of critical safety information across borders.

Understanding CIOMS principles is essential for pharmacovigilance professionals operating in global environments. These guidelines facilitate harmonization across regulatory jurisdictions, ensuring consistent safety standards while accommodating regional differences. As pharmacovigilance continues evolving, CIOMS working groups will address emerging challenges including real-world evidence integration, artificial intelligence applications, and patient-centric safety monitoring.

CHAPTER 16

CDSCO (INDIA) AND PHARMACOVIGILANCE

KEY OUTCOMES

Upon completion of this chapter, learners will be able to:

1. Understand CDSCO structure, functions, and regulatory authority
2. Explain key provisions of Drugs and Cosmetics Act 1940 and Rules 1945
3. Describe Schedule Y requirements for clinical trials in India
4. Apply New Drugs and Clinical Trials Rules 2019
5. Understand PvPI structure and ADR reporting in India
6. Compare Indian and global pharmacovigilance requirements
7. Recognize harmonization efforts with FDA, EMA, and MHRA

ABSTRACT

The Central Drugs Standard Control Organization (CDSCO) serves as India's national regulatory authority for pharmaceuticals and medical devices. Operating under the Directorate General of Health Services, CDSCO ensures safety, efficacy, and quality of drugs marketed in India. This chapter examines CDSCO's structure and functions, the legislative framework provided by the Drugs and Cosmetics Act 1940 and Rules 1945, Schedule Y requirements for clinical trials, the New Drugs and Clinical Trials Rules 2019, and India's national pharmacovigilance infrastructure through the Pharmacovigilance Programme of India (PvPI). Understanding Indian regulatory requirements and their alignment with global standards is essential for professionals working in India's pharmaceutical sector or conducting clinical research in Indian populations.

16.1 CENTRAL DRUGS STANDARD CONTROL ORGANIZATION (CDSCO)

The Central Drugs Standard Control Organization (CDSCO) is India's national regulatory authority responsible for ensuring safety, efficacy, and quality of pharmaceuticals, biologicals, and medical devices. Headquartered in New Delhi, CDSCO operates under the Ministry of Health and Family Welfare, Directorate General of Health Services.

CDSCO's primary mandates include approval of new drugs and clinical trials, regulation of imported drugs, standardization and quality control of pharmaceuticals, coordination with State Drug Control Organizations, and supervision of pharmacovigilance activities through the National Coordination Centre for Pharmacovigilance Programme of India.

The organization works in collaboration with state drug regulatory authorities, which enforce the Drugs and Cosmetics Act at the state level, inspect manufacturing facilities, and monitor drug quality within their jurisdictions.

16.2 STRUCTURE AND FUNCTIONS OF CDSCO

Organizational Structure:

CDSCO is headed by the Drugs Controller General of India (DCGI), who serves as the chief drug regulatory authority. The organization comprises several divisions including New Drugs Division (approves new drugs and clinical trials), Biological Division (regulates vaccines and blood products), Medical Devices Division (oversees medical device regulation), Import Division (controls drug imports), Pharmacovigilance Division (coordinates PvPI), and Zonal and Port Offices (inspect imports and manufacturing facilities).

Key Functions:

Regulatory approval: CDSCO reviews applications for marketing authorization of new drugs, biologicals, and medical devices. The approval process includes evaluation of safety, efficacy, and quality data.

Clinical trial approval: All clinical trials in India require CDSCO permission. The organization reviews trial protocols for scientific validity, ethical compliance, and patient safety provisions.

Import regulation: Imported drugs require registration and testing certificates from CDSCO port offices before distribution in India.

Standards setting: CDSCO establishes quality standards for pharmaceuticals in coordination with the Indian Pharmacopoeia Commission.

Inspection and enforcement: CDSCO conducts inspections of manufacturing facilities applying for new drug approvals and coordinates with state authorities for enforcement actions.

Pharmacovigilance coordination: Through the National Coordination Centre, CDSCO oversees India's pharmacovigilance infrastructure, collects adverse event reports, and coordinates safety communications.

16.3 DRUGS AND COSMETICS ACT, 1940

The Drugs and Cosmetics Act, 1940 is the primary legislation regulating manufacture, import, distribution, and sale of drugs and cosmetics in India. The Act provides legal framework for drug regulation and establishes penalties for violations.

Key Provisions:

Definitions (Section 3): Defines drugs, new drugs, Ayurvedic/Unani/Siddha drugs, and cosmetics. A "new drug" includes drugs not previously used in India, new indications, new dosage forms, and drugs used for different patient populations.

Prohibition of manufacture and sale (Sections 18-18D): Prohibits manufacture, sale, or distribution of drugs without valid license, substandard drugs, misbranded or adulterated drugs, and drugs not conforming to prescribed standards.

Central and State Drug Authorities (Sections 21-33): Establishes central and state drug control authorities, defines their powers and functions, and provides for appointment of drug inspectors.

Licensing (Sections 18A-18E): Requires licenses for manufacturing, sale, and distribution. Specifies conditions for license issuance and suspension or cancellation procedures.

Import regulations (Section 10): Empowers government to prohibit import of drugs not conforming to Indian standards or quality requirements.

Penalties (Sections 27-28): Prescribes punishment for violations including imprisonment and fines for manufacturing or selling substandard, adulterated, or spurious drugs.

16.4 DRUGS AND COSMETICS RULES, 1945

The Drugs and Cosmetics Rules, 1945 provide detailed regulations for implementing the Drugs and Cosmetics Act. The Rules specify technical requirements, procedures, and standards for drug regulation.

Important Schedules:

Schedule C: Lists biological and special products requiring specific manufacturing standards.

Schedule M: Prescribes Good Manufacturing Practices (GMP) for pharmaceutical manufacturing facilities.

Schedule Y: Details requirements for conducting clinical trials and import of new drugs for clinical research.

Schedule X: Lists drugs requiring special storage, sale, and prescription requirements.

Schedule H: Specifies prescription-only medicines.

Schedule G: Lists drugs requiring warning labels on dispensing.

The Rules establish licensing procedures, specify application formats and fees, define manufacturing standards, prescribe labeling requirements, and outline procedures for import and export.

Amendments to the Rules allow CDSCO to update regulatory requirements without parliamentary legislation, enabling timely responses to evolving pharmaceutical landscape.

16.5 SCHEDULE Y REQUIREMENTS

Schedule Y of the Drugs and Cosmetics Rules govern clinical trial requirements in India. Originally introduced in 1988 and substantially revised in 2005 and 2019, Schedule Y aligns Indian clinical trial regulations with international standards while addressing India-specific considerations.

Key Requirements:

Ethics Committee Approval: All clinical trials require approval from registered Ethics Committees following ICH-GCP guidelines. Ethics Committees must include independent members, medical experts, legal experts, and social scientists.

Informed Consent: Written informed consent is mandatory in language understandable to participants. Consent process must explain trial purpose, procedures, risks, benefits, and voluntary nature.

Clinical Trial Phases: Schedule Y recognizes standard trial phases (I, II, III, IV) and specifies requirements for each. Phase I trials typically require healthy volunteers except for oncology and life-threatening conditions.

New Drug Applications: For global new drugs (not approved anywhere), complete clinical data including Indian clinical trials may be required. For drugs approved in ICH countries, limited Indian bridging studies may suffice.

Pharmacovigilance: Sponsors must establish pharmacovigilance systems, report serious adverse events within specified timelines (7-14 days), and submit periodic safety reports.

Compensation: Schedule Y mandates compensation for trial-related injuries or deaths. Compensation amount depends on severity and permanent disability degree.

16.6 NEW DRUGS AND CLINICAL TRIALS RULES, 2019

The New Drugs and Clinical Trials Rules, 2019 replaced earlier Schedule Y provisions, modernizing India's clinical trial regulatory framework. The Rules aim to facilitate clinical research while strengthening patient safety and ethical oversight.

Major Changes:

Centralized online system: Clinical trial applications are submitted through CDSCO's online portal, improving transparency and processing efficiency. The system provides timelines for regulatory review and approval.

Risk-based categorization: Clinical trials are categorized based on risk levels. Low-risk studies receive faster approval, while high-risk trials undergo detailed review.

Timelines for approval: CDSCO must respond within specified timeframes (90 days for new applications). Deemed approval provisions apply if timelines are not met.

Waiver of local trials: For drugs approved in developed markets with adequate safety data, requirement for Indian clinical trials may be waived based on scientific justification.

Audio-visual recording: Informed consent process must be documented through audio-visual recording, ensuring proper consent procedures.

Compensation provisions: Detailed compensation guidelines specify amounts based on injury severity. No-fault compensation is provided for trial-related injuries regardless of causality.

Post-trial access: Sponsors must provide post-trial access to investigational products for trial participants who benefited, ensuring continuity of care.

16.7 PHARMACOVIGILANCE PROGRAMME OF INDIA (PvPI) STRUCTURE

The Pharmacovigilance Programme of India (PvPI) is the national program for monitoring drug safety, established in 2010 under CDSCO. PvPI collects, analyzes, and disseminates information on adverse drug reactions to ensure patient safety.

Structure:

National Coordination Centre (NCC-PvPI): Located at Indian Pharmacopoeia Commission, Ghaziabad, the NCC serves as the national hub. Functions include collecting ADR reports from across India, maintaining national ADR database, analyzing safety signals, coordinating with WHO-UMC Uppsala, conducting causality assessment, and disseminating safety alerts.

Regional Centres: PvPI has established multiple Regional Pharmacovigilance Centers at major medical institutions across India. These centers coordinate pharmacovigilance activities within their regions, train healthcare professionals, promote ADR reporting, and provide technical support to peripheral centers.

Peripheral Centres: Peripheral centers, typically located at district hospitals and medical colleges, collect ADR reports from healthcare facilities, verify report completeness, conduct initial causality assessment, and transmit reports to regional centers.

ADR Monitoring Centres (AMCs): AMCs are healthcare facilities enrolled in PvPI that actively report ADRs. India has over 300 AMCs distributed across states.

16.8 NATIONAL COORDINATION CENTRE (NCC-PvPI)

The National Coordination Centre for Pharmacovigilance Programme of India (NCC-PvPI) serves as the apex body coordinating all pharmacovigilance activities in India. Established at the Indian Pharmacopoeia Commission, Ghaziabad, the NCC operates under CDSCO's regulatory oversight.

Key Functions:

Database management: The NCC maintains VigiFlow, India's national ADR database compatible with WHO's VigiBase. All ADR reports are entered, coded using MedDRA and WHO-DD, and transmitted to WHO-UMC.

Signal detection: Regular data mining and statistical analysis identify potential safety signals. Signals are evaluated for clinical significance and public health impact.

Causality assessment: The NCC conducts causality assessment using WHO-UMC scale and Naranjo algorithm, determining likelihood that reported adverse events are drug-related.

Safety communication: The NCC issues safety alerts, drug safety newsletters, and updates to healthcare professionals about emerging safety concerns.

Training and capacity building: Regular training programs for healthcare professionals promote ADR awareness and reporting culture. E-learning modules and educational materials are developed.

International collaboration: As WHO Programme member, India shares safety data internationally and participates in global signal detection activities.

16.9 ADR REPORTING FORMAT IN INDIA

India uses standardized ADR reporting forms aligned with international formats. The PvPI ADR reporting form captures essential information for causality assessment and signal detection.

Form Sections:

Patient details: Age, gender, patient identification number (maintaining confidentiality), weight, relevant medical history, and known allergies.

Adverse reaction details: Description of reaction(s), onset date and time, severity (mild, moderate, severe), seriousness criteria (death, life-threatening, hospitalization, disability, congenital anomaly), and outcome (recovered, recovering, not recovered, fatal, unknown).

Suspected medication(s): Drug name (generic and brand), dose, route, frequency, indication for use, therapy start and stop dates, and action taken (drug withdrawn, dose reduced, continued).

Concomitant medications: Other drugs taken by patient with doses and therapy dates.

Relevant investigations: Laboratory data, diagnostic tests, biopsy findings relevant to the adverse event.

Dechallenge and rechallenge: Information if drug was stopped and reaction subsided (dechallenge) or restarted and reaction recurred (rechallenge).

Reporter information: Reporter name, designation, contact details, institution, and reporting date.

Reports can be submitted online through PvPI portal, by email, by post, or through mobile application (PvPI-ADR application). Healthcare professionals, patients, and pharmaceutical companies can submit reports.

16.10 DIFFERENCES IN INDIAN AND GLOBAL PHARMACOVIGILANCE REQUIREMENTS

While India has harmonized many pharmacovigilance requirements with international standards, some differences exist:

Reporting timelines: India follows similar timelines as ICH (15 days for serious expected, 7 days for serious unexpected ADRs). However, specific reporting requirements for PSURs differ from EU-PSUR cycles.

Causality assessment: India emphasizes causality assessment using WHO-UMC scale, whereas some regions rely more on narrative descriptions.

Compensation provisions: India's clinical trial compensation requirements are more prescriptive, and mandatory compared to many Western countries.

PSUR requirements: India requires PSURs at 6-month intervals for first two years post-approval, annually for next two years, then every five years. EU follows product-specific PSUR cycles.

Language: ADR reports and regulatory submissions in India must be in English, whereas EU accepts multiple languages.

Periodic benefit-risk evaluation reports (PBRERs): India is transitioning from traditional PSURs to ICH-E2C(R2) format PBRERs, but implementation is gradual.

Risk Management Plans: While India encourages RMPs, they are not mandatory for all products unlike EU requirements.

16.11 COMPARISON WITH FDA, EMA, MHRA REQUIREMENTS

Table 27: Comparison of Key Pharmacovigilance Requirements

Aspect	India (CDSCO)	USA (FDA)	EU (EMA)	UK (MHRA)
Serious ADR Reporting	15 days for expected, 7 days for unexpected	15 days for ICSRs	15 days for serious ADRs	15 days for serious ADRs
Periodic Reports	PSUR (transitioning to PBER)	Annual reports for NDAs	PSUR/PBRER as per EURD list	PSUR/PBRER aligned with EU
Risk Management Plans	Encouraged, not mandatory for all	REMS for specific products	Mandatory for all new products	Mandatory, aligned with EU

Signal Detection	Required, methodology evolving	Mandatory with defined processes	Mandatory with EudraVigilance	Mandatory with Yellow Card
QPPV Requirement	Not explicitly required	Not required	Mandatory	Mandatory
PSMF	Not required	Not required	Mandatory	Mandatory

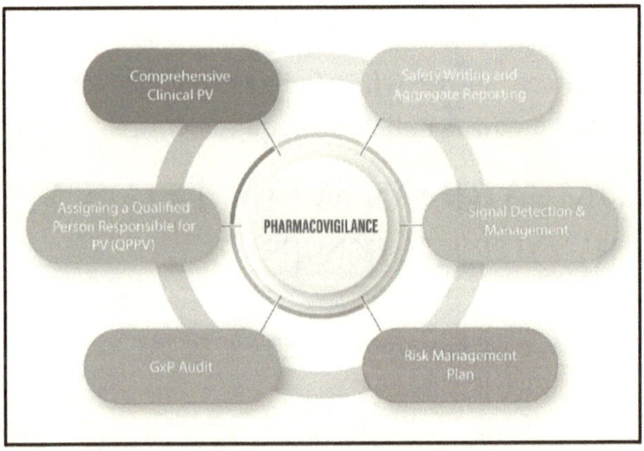

Figure 19: This table compares key pharmacovigilance requirements across major regulatory jurisdictions, highlighting areas of harmonization and differences that multinational pharmaceutical companies must navigate.

Key Similarities:

All jurisdictions require timely reporting of serious adverse events, follow ICH-E2A definitions of seriousness, use standardized terminologies (MedDRA), participate in international signal detection, and emphasize patient safety as primary objective.

Key Differences:

Regulatory infrastructure: EU requires QPPV and PSMF; India and FDA do not. Periodic reporting: Different cycles and formats across regions. Risk management: EU has most stringent RMP requirements; India is developing framework. Database access: FDA has FAERS public database; India's database is restricted.

16.12 REGULATORY HARMONIZATION EFFORTS

India is actively pursuing regulatory harmonization with international standards to facilitate drug development and ensure patient safety.

ICH Membership: India became an ICH member in 2018, committing to implement ICH guidelines. Implementation of ICH-E2A through E2F guidelines for pharmacovigilance is underway.

PSUR to PBRER Transition: India is transitioning from traditional PSUR format to ICH-E2C(R2) PBRER format, aligning with global standards.

MedDRA Adoption: India uses MedDRA for adverse event coding, facilitating international data exchange.

WHO Programme: As WHO Programme member since 1997, India contributes to and benefits from global safety data sharing.

Bilateral Cooperation: CDSCO has established collaborative agreements with FDA, EMA, MHRA, and other regulators for information exchange and regulatory convergence.

Challenges in Harmonization:

Different legal frameworks, resource constraints for implementing complex systems, need to balance international standards with local healthcare context, capacity building requirements for regulatory staff, and infrastructure development for electronic reporting systems.

Despite challenges, harmonization efforts continue strengthening India's pharmacovigilance system while maintaining regulatory sovereignty and addressing India-specific public health needs.

CDSCO plays a central role in safeguarding Indian patients through comprehensive drug regulation and pharmacovigilance oversight. The Drugs and Cosmetics Act and Rules provide robust legal framework, while Schedule Y and Clinical Trials Rules establish standards for ethical research. The Pharmacovigilance Programme of India has created nationwide infrastructure for ADR monitoring, with the National Coordination Centre serving as the data hub.

India's pharmacovigilance system continues maturing, with ongoing harmonization with ICH guidelines and international best practices. Understanding both Indian regulatory requirements and global standards is essential for pharmaceutical professionals operating in India's dynamic healthcare environment. As India strengthens its pharmacovigilance capabilities, it contributes increasingly to global drug safety knowledge while protecting its population.

Appendix

APPENDIX – 1

Suspected ADR Reporting Format – IPC

The Indian Pharmacopoeia Commission (IPC) coordinates the Pharmacovigilance Programme of India (PvPI), which mandates the systematic documentation of suspected adverse drug reactions (ADRs) by healthcare professionals. The dedicated IPC form collects essential details, including patient demographics, a brief description of the adverse event, medication(s) involved, onset date, medical history, and concomitant therapies. These forms are accessible online via the IPC website or from local Adverse Drug Reaction Monitoring Centers (AMCs) and can be submitted by post, email, or toll-free number. The PvPI encourages the reporting of all types of ADRs, whether minor or severe, facilitating Indian pharmacovigilance and medicine safety through continuous data monitoring and analysis.

APPENDIX

Version-1.3

SUSPECTED ADVERSE DRUG REACTION REPORTING FORM

For VOLUNTARY reporting of Adverse Drug Reaction by Healthcare Professionals

INDIAN PHARMACOPOEIA COMMISSION(National Coordination Centre-Pharmacovigilance Programme of India)

Ministry of Health & Family Welfare, Government of India Sector-23, Raj Nagar, Ghaziabad-201002

A. PATIENT INFORMATION			Reg. No. /IPD No. /OPD No. /CR No. :
1. Patient Initials ______	2. Age at the time of Event or Date of Birth ________	3. M ☐ F ☐ Other ☐	AMC Report No. :
		4. Weight______Kgs	Worldwide Unique No. :

B. SUSPECTED ADVERSE REACTION

5. Event/Reaction start date (dd/mm/yyyy)

6. Event/Reaction stop date (dd/mm/yyyy)

6 (A). Onset Lag Time

7. Describe Event/Reaction with treatment details, if any

12. Relevant tests/ laboratory data with dates

13. Relevant medical/medication history (e.g. allergies, race, pregnancy, smoking, alcohol use, hepatic/renal dysfunction, past surgery etc.)

14. Seriousness of the reaction: No ☐ if Yes ☐(please tick anyone)

☐ Death (dd/mm/yyyy) ☐ Congenital-anomaly

☐ Life threatening ☐ Disability

☐Hospitalization/Prolonged ☐ Other Medically important

15. Outcomes

☐ Recovered ☐ Recovering ☐ Not recovered

☐ Fatal ☐ Recovered with sequelae ☐ Unknown

C. SUSPECTED MEDICATION(S)

S.No	8. Name (Brand/Generic)	Manufacturer (if known)	Batch No. / Lot No.	Exp. Date (if known)	Dose used	Route used	Frequency (OD, BD etc.)	Therapy dates: Date started	Therapy dates: Date stopped	Indication	Causality Assessment
i											
ii											
iii											
iv*											

S.No as per C	9. Action Taken (please tick): Drug withdrawn	Dose increased	Dose reduced	Dose not changed	Not applicable	Unknown	10. Reaction reappeared after reintroduction (please tick): Yes	No	Effect unknown	Dose (if reintroduced)
i										
ii										
iii										
iv										

11. Concomitant medical product including self-medication and herbal remedies with therapy dates (Exclude those used to treat reaction)

S.No	Name (Brand/Generic)	Dose used	Route used	Frequency (OD, BD, etc.)	Therapy dates: Date started	Therapy dates: Date stopped	Indication
i							
ii							
iii*							

Additional Information:

D. REPORTER DETAILS

16. Name and Professional Address:____________________

____

Pin:__________E-mail____________________

Tel. No. (with STD code)____________________

Occupation:______________ Signature:______________

17. Date of this report (dd/mm/yyyy):

Sig. and Name of Receiver-

Confidentiality: The patient's identity is held in strict confidence and protected to the fullest extent. Submission of a report does not constitute an admission that medical personnel or manufacturer or the product caused or contributed to the reaction. Submission of an ADR report does not have any legal implication on the reporter.

*use separate page for more information

National Coordination Centre for Pharmacovigilance Programme of India
Ministry of Health & Family Welfare, Government of India
Sector-23, Raj Nagar, Ghaziabad-201002
Tel.: 0120-2783400, 2783401, 2783392, Fax: 0120-2783311
www.ipc.nic.in

ADVICE ABOUT REPORTING

A. What to report?

- Report serious adverse drug reactions. A reaction is serious when the patient outcome is:
  - Death
  - Life-threatening
  - Hospitalization (initial or prolonged)
  - Disability (significant, persistent or permanent)
  - Congenital anomaly
  - Required intervention to prevent permanent impairment or damage
- Report non-serious, known or unknown, frequent or rare adverse drug reactions due to Medicines, Vaccines and Herbal products etc.

Note- Adverse Event Following Immunization can also be reported in Serious AEFI case Notification Form available on http://www.ipc.gov.in**)**

B. Who can report?

- All healthcare professionals (Clinicians, Dentists, Pharmacists and Nurses etc) can report adverse drug reactions

C. Where to report?

- Duly filled inSuspected Adverse Drug Reaction Reporting Form can be sent to the nearest Adverse Drug Reaction Monitoring Centre (AMC) or directly to the National Coordination Centre (NCC) for PvPI.
- Call on Helpline (Toll Free) 1800 180 3024 to report ADRs or directly mail this filled form to pvpi.ipc@gov.in
- A list of nationwide AMCs is available at:
  http://www.ipc.gov.in, http://www.ipc.gov.in/PvPI/pv_home.html

D. What happens to the submitted information?

- Information provided in this form is handled in strict confidence. The causality assessment is carried out at AMCs by using WHO-UMC scale. The analyzed forms are forwarded to the NCC through ADR database. Finally the data is analyzed and forwarded to the Global Pharmacovigilance Database managed by WHO Uppsala Monitoring Centre in Sweden.
- The reports are periodically reviewed by the NCC-PvPI. The information generated on the basis of these reports helps in continuous assessment of the benefit-risk ratio of medicines.
- The Signal Review Panel of PvPI to review the data and suggest any interventions that may be required.

E. Mandatory fields for suspected ADR reporting form

- Patient initials, age at onset of reaction, reaction term(s), date of onset of reaction, suspected medication(s) and reporter information.

For ADRs Reporting

- **E-mail:** pvpi.ipc@gov.in
- ***PvPI Helpline (Toll Free):*** *1800 180 3024(9:00 AM to 5:30 PM, Monday-Friday)*
- ***ADR Mobile App: "ADR PvPI"***

APPENDIX - 2

Adverse Reaction Due to Blood Transfusion – Haemovigilance Program of India

The Haemovigilance Programme of India, managed by the National Institute of Biologicals (NIB), provides comprehensive formats for capturing adverse transfusion reactions in recipients and donors. Adverse events, such as febrile reactions, allergic responses, hemolytic reactions, and transfusion-transmitted infections, are documented using the official Transfusion Reaction Reporting Form (TRRF), which requests detailed clinical data, product specificity, dates, and possible causes of the adverse events. Additionally, donor reaction reporting forms gather data on events that occur during donation. Data were uploaded to the Haemo-Vigil software for review and analysis, which collectively supports improved transfusion safety and clinical practices nationwide.

APPENDIX

National Institute of Biologicals

Ministry of Health & Family Welfare, Govt. of India

(National Coordinating Center)

HAEMOVIGILANCE PROGRAMME OF INDIA

Transfusion Reaction Reporting Form (TRRF) For Blood & Blood Components & Plasma Products (Version-2)

* Mandatory Field

(A) Patient Information

Hospital Code No.:						
Patient Initials*:	Gender*:	Blood Group*:				
Hospital Admission No.*:	Age/Date of Birth*:	.......Yrs	.......Month	......Days	......Hrs	..........Mins
Primary Diagnosis*:						
Medical History:						

(B) Transfusion Reaction Details*

Was the patient under anaesthesia during transfusion: Yes/No if Yes type : GA/Spinal/LA

	Temp:	Pulse:	BP:	RR:	SPO2:
Pre-transfusion Vitals:	Temp:	Pulse:	BP:	RR:	SPO2:
Vitals at the time of reaction:	Temp:	Pulse:	BP:	RR:	SPO2:

Please tick mark the relevant signs and symptoms listed below

Generalised		Pain	Respiratory	Renal	Circulatory
☐ Fever	☐ Anxiety	☐ Chest Pain	☐ Dyspnoea	☐ Haematuria	☐ Tachycardia
☐ Chills	☐ Itching (Pruritus)	☐ Abdominal	☐ Wheeze	☐ Haemoglobinuria	☐ Hypertension
☐ Rigors	☐ Edema (Site)___	☐ Back/Flank Pain	☐ Cough	☐ Oliguria	☐ Hypotension
☐ Nausea	☐ Juandice	☐ Infusion Site Pain	☐ Hypoxemia	☐ Other_____	☐ Raised JVP
☐ Urticaria	☐ Other_____	☐ Other_____	☐ Bilateral Infiltrates on Chest X-ray		☐ Arrhythmias
☐ Flushing					☐ Other_____
☐ Restlessness					
☐ Vomiting			☐ Other_____		

Any Other(Specify) : ....

(C) Transfusion Product(s) Details*

Select*	Select Component	Select Indication	Date & Time of Issue of Blood Component	Date & Time of onset Transfusion	Unit Id (Transfused)	Blood Group	Volume Transfused (ml)	Expiry date of Blood Component	Manufacturer of Blood Bag	Batch / Lot No. of the Blood Bag	1st time/ repeat Transfusion
☐	Whole blood										
☐	Packed Red blood cells (PRBC)										☐ 1st Time
☐	Buffy coat depleted PRBC										
☐	Leucofiltered PRBC										
☐	Random Donor platelets/ pooled										☐ Repeat 1 to 10
☐	Apheresis Platelets										
☐	Fresh Frozen Plasma										☐ Repeat > 10
☐	Cryoprecipitate										
☐	Any Other										

Add New Plasma Product

Select	Plasma Product	Indication	Date of Administration	Manufacturer	Expiry Date of the Plasma Product	Batch No. / Lot No.	1st Time / Repeat
							☐ 1st Time ☐ Repeat 1 to 10 ☐ Repeat > 10

APPENDIX

(D) Investigations

	Clerical Checks	Specify Error Found if any: ______	
	Investigation	**Pre-transfusion sample**	**Post-transfusion sample**
☐	Visual Check		
* ☐	Repeat Blood Grouping	O+ /A+ /B+ /AB+ /O- /A- /B- /AB-	O+ /A+ /B+ /AB+ /O- /A- /B- /AB-
* ☐	Repeat Crossmatch	☐ Compatible ☐ InCompatible ☐ Not Done	☐ Compatible ☐ InCompatible ☐ Not Done
* ☐	Repeat Antibody screen	☐ Negative ☐ Positive ☐ Not Done	☐ Negative ☐ Positive ☐ Not Done
☐	Antibody Identification		
* ☐	Direct antiglobulin test	☐ Negative ☐ Positive ☐ Not Done	☐ Negative ☐ Positive ☐ Not Done
☐	Hemoglobin		
☐	Plasma Hemoglobin		
☐	Urine hemoglobin		
☐	Bilirubin (Total/conjugated)		
☐	Platelet count		
☐	PT/INR		
* ☐	Blood culture of Blood Bag	☐ Negative ☐ Positive ☐ Not Done	Specify Organism if positive______
* ☐	Blood culture of Patient	☐ Negative ☐ Positive ☐ Not Done Specify Organism if positive______	☐ Negative ☐ Positive ☐ Not Done Specify Organism if positive______
☐	Chest X-ray of the patient in case of suspected TRALI		

In case of Non-immune hemolysis (which of the following was the case?)

☐	Hemolysis due to freezing of PRBC Units
☐	Hemolysis due to inappropriate warming of PRBC Units
☐	Hemolysis due to infusion of any other fluid through same BT set. Specify Fluid:______
☐	Mechanical damage

In Case of ABO Mismatch (which of the following was the case?)

☐	Wrong Blood in tube
☐	Grouping error
☐	Labelling error
☐	Wrong unit transfused

(E) Nature of Adverse Reaction(s)*

Select	Reaction	Date & Time of Onset of Reaction	Date & Time of Recovery	Outcome
☐	Febrile Non Haemolytic Reactions (FNHTR) 1° C rise in temperature ☐ 2° C rise in temperature ☐ Only Chills & Rigors ☐			☐ 1. Death following the Adverse Reaction(s)
☐	Allergic reaction			
☐	Anaphylaxis			
☐	Immunological Haemolysis due to ABO Incompatibility			
☐	Immunological Haemolysis due to other Allo-Antibodies			
☐	Non Immunological Haemolysis			☐ 2. Recovered
☐	Hypotensive Transfusion Reaction			
☐	Transfusion Related Acute Lung Injury (TRALI) Definite ☐ Possible ☐			
☐	Transfusion Associated Dyspnoea (TAD)			☐ 3. Recovered with Sequelae
☐	Transfusion Associated Circulatory Overload (TACO)			
☐	Transfusion Transmitted Bacterial Infection			
☐	Transfusion Transmitted Parasitic Infection (Malaria)			
☐	Post Transfusion Purpura			
☐	Transfusion Associated Graft versus Host Disease (TAGvHD)			☐ 4. Unknown
☐	Other Reaction (s) Add New			

IMPUTABILITY ASSESSMENT

(F) Imputability Assessment*

S. No.	Reaction Term	Transfusion Product/ Component	*Imputability Assessment (Please mention from the below list)

*Imputability: 1. Definite (Certain), 2. Probable (Likely), 3. Possible, 4. Unlikely (Doubtful), 5. Excluded, 6. Not Assessed

Monthly Denominator Reporting Form

Hospital Code :	Month/Year:
Blood Component	**No.of Units Issued**
1) Fresh Frozen Plasma	
2) Whole Blood	
3) Packed Red Blood Cells (PRBC)	
4) Buffy Coat Depleted PRBC	
5) Leucofiltered PRBC	
6) Random Donor Platelets/ Pooled	
7) Apheresis Platelets	
8) Cryoprecipitate	
9) Any Other______	

APPENDIX - 3

Medical Device Adverse Event Reporting Form (MvPI) India

Under the Materiovigilance Programme of India (MvPI), the adverse event reporting system for medical devices employs a standardized form to log any device-related hazards, malfunctions, or user errors that result in patient harm or risk. This reporting template requires information such as device identification and batch numbers, classification (risk category), a thorough event narrative, patient details, and the role of the user and manufacturer. Confidentiality is assured with the aim of detecting unsafe trends and initiating corrective regulatory actions. Reports can be made by users, healthcare institutes, distributors and manufacturers through official IPC channels.

APPENDIX

MEDICAL DEVICE ADVERSE EVENT REPORTING FORM

Materiovigilance Programme of India (MvPI)

This form is intended to collect information on Medical Devices Adverse Event in India. The form is designed to be used voluntarily by Manufacturer/Importer/Distributor of Medical Devices, Healthcare Professionals and anyone with direct/indirect knowledge of Medical Devices Adverse Event.

General Information

1. Date of Report :
2. Type of Report : Initial ☐ Follow up ☐ Final ☐ Trend ☐
3. Reporter Reference for MDMC only: • Centre • Location • Month-Year • Case No.

Reporter Details

1. Type of Reporter : (a) Manufacturer ☐ (b) Importer ☐ (c) Distributor ☐ (d) Healthcare Professional ☐
   (e) Patient ☐ (f) Others ☐ specify ....
2. In case, where the reporter is not manufacturer, fill the following details:-
   (a) Has the reporter informed the incident to the manufacturer?
   Yes ☐ No ☐
   (b) Is the reporter also submitting the report on behalf of the manufacturer?
   Yes ☐ No ☐
3. Reporter contact information:
   a) Name :
   b) Address :
   c) Tel. /Mobile :
   d) Email :

Device Category

Medical Device	In Vitro Diagnostics (IVD)	Medical Equipments / Machines
I. Therapeutic ☐ Diagnostic ☐	I. Kits ☐	I. Therapeutic ☐ Diagnostic ☐
Both ☐ Preventive ☐	II. Reagents ☐	II. Therapeutic & Diagnostic ☐
Assistive ☐	III. Calibrator ☐	III. Preventive ☐
II. Implantable device ☐	IV. Control Material ☐	IV. Assistive ☐
Non-Implantable device ☐	V. Others ☐	V. Imaging ☐
III. Invasive ☐ Non-Invasive ☐	VI. IVD electronic reader/ Analyzer ☐	VI. Invasive ☐ Non-Invasive ☐
IV. Single use device ☐		VII. Others ☐
Reusable device ☐		
Reuse of manufacture marked Single use device ☐		
V. Sterile ☐ Non Sterile ☐		
VI. Personal use / Homecare use ☐		

Instruction for use Section A-F

- ***If Medical Devices/Equipments/Machines : Please fill all the sections i.e. A, B, C, D, E & F***
- ***If in Vitro Diagnostics (IVD) : Please fill sections i.e. A (except 6, 7, 8, 13, 14 & 16), B (except 1, 2, 6 & 8), D, E, & F***

APPENDIX

(A) Device Details

Device Name / Trade Name / Brand Name: ....

Details	Name	Address
Manufacturer		
Importer		
Distributor		

1. a) Is the device notified/regulated in India : Yes ☐ No ☐

   b) Device Risk Classification as per India MDR 2017 : A ☐ B ☐ C ☐ D ☐

2. License No. (Manufacture/Import) :
3. Catalogue No. :
4. Model No. :
5. Lot / Batch No. :
6. Serial No. :
7. Software Version :
8. Associated Devices / Accessories :
9. Nomenclature Code if applicable; GMDN/UMDNS :
10. UDI No. (If applicable) :
11. Installation Date :
12. Expiration Date :
13. Last preventive maintenance date (dd/mm/yyyy) :
14. Last calibration date (dd/mm/yyyy) :
15. Year of manufacturing :
16. How long was device/Equipment/Machine in use :
17. Availability of device for evaluation : Yes ☐ No ☐

    If no, was the device destroyed ☐ Still in use ☐ return to manufacturer or importer/distributor ☐

18. Is the usage of device as per manufacturer claim /Instruction for use/user manual: Yes ☐ No ☐

    If no specify usage ....

    ....

19. For devices not regulated / notified in India : Regulator / Regulatory status in country of origin

    ....

APPENDIX

(B) Event Description

1. Date of Event / Near miss incident:
2. Date of Implant/Explant (If applicable):
3. Location of Event:
   Hospital Premise ☐ Manufacture/Distributor premise ☐
   Home ☐ Others ☐
4. Device Operator:-
   Healthcare Professional ☐ Patient ☐ Others ☐
   Problem noted prior to use/near miss event ☐
5. Device disposition / Current location:
   a) Returned to company ☐ If yes, date ....../....... /.......
   b) Remains implanted in patient ☐
   c) Within the healthcare facility ☐
   d) At patient home ☐
   e) Destroyed ☐
   f) Others (specify) ☐
6. Is device in use after incidence : Yes ☐ No ☐

7. Serious event: ☐
   If serious, Tick the appropriate reason
   a) Death (DD/MM/YY) ☐ ..../............/............
   b) Life Threatening ☐
   c) Disability or permanent damage ☐
   d) Hospitalization ☐
   e) Congenital anomaly /birth defect ☐
   f) Any other serious (Imp. medical event) ☐
   g) Required intervention to prevent / permanent Impairment / damage device ☐
8. Non serious event ☐
9. Whether other medical devices were used at same time with above device if yes, please specify name(s)/use(s)
   ....
   ....
   ....

10. Detail description of Event:-

For manufacturer/authorized representative use only

11. Frequency of occurrence of similar Adverse Event in India in past 3 years	Year	No. of Similar Adverse Events	Total No. Supplied	Frequency of Occurrence (%)

12. Frequency of occurrence of similar Adverse Event in globally in past 3 years	Year	No. of Similar Adverse Events	Total No. Supplied	Frequency of Occurrence (%)

(C) Patient Information, History & Outcome

1. Patient Hospital ID :
2. Patient Initial :
3. Age :
4. Gender : Male ☐ Female ☐ Others ☐
5. Weight :
6. Other relevant history, including pre-existing medical conditions..
   ....
   ....
   ....
   ....

7. Patient Outcomes:
   a) Recovered Date (DD/MM/YY) ☐ ....../......./.......
   b) Not yet recovered ☐
   c) Death ☐ (DD/MM/YY) ☐ ....../......./.......
   d) Others ☐
   Please specify..
   ....
   ....
   ....
   ....
   ....

(D) Healthcare Facility Information (if available)

1. Name :
2. Address :
3. Contact Person Name at the site of event :
4. Tel. No. :

(E) Causality Assessment

1. Investigation action taken:
2. Root cause of problem (Applicable for follow up / final reports):

(F) Manufacturer/Authorized Representative Investigation & Action taken

1. Manufacturer/Authorized Representative device risk analysis report:
2. Corrective / preventive action taken:
3. Device history review:

Where to report?

Duly filled Medical Device Adverse Event Reporting Form can be sent to Indian Pharmacopoeia Commission, Ministry of Health and Family Welfare, Government of India, Sector-23, Rajnagar, Ghaziabad 20002, Tel 0120-2783400, 2783401 and 2783392, FAX:0120-2783311 or email to mvpi.ipcindia@gmail.com **Or Call on Helpline no. 1800 180 3024 to report Adverse event.**

Partnering Organizations

Disclaimer

Confidentiality: The patient's identity is held in strict confidence and protected to the fullest extent. Programme staff is not expected to and will not disclose the reporter's identity in response to a request from the public. Submission of a report does not constitute an admission that medical personnel or manufacturer or the product caused or contributed to the adverse event.

APPENDIX – 4

Vaccine Adverse Event Reporting Form - India

India's Adverse Event Following Immunization (AEFI) program mandates standardized forms for reporting vaccine-related adverse events, regardless of severity. The primary reporting format collects recipient information and vaccination details, with specific fields for the nature, onset, and outcome of the event. Healthcare workers must report serious or severe AEFIs within 24 h, escalating through district and national committees for expert evaluation and timely intervention. The system supports the continuous safety monitoring of all vaccines used under the Universal Immunization Program and the private sector.

APPENDIX

AEFI reporting ID number:

REPORTING FORM FOR ADVERSE EVENTS FOLLOWING IMMUNIZATION (AEFI)

Patient Name:	***Reporter's Name:***
Patient's full Address:	Institution:
	Designation & Department:
Telephone:	Address:
Sex: ☐ M ☐ F	
Date of birth : __/__/__	Telephone & E-mail:
OR Age at onset: ☐☐ *Years* ☐☐ *Months* ☐☐☐ *Days*	Date patient notified event to health system: __/__/__
OR Age Group at onset: ☐ *<1 Year* ☐ *1 to 5 Years* ☐ *>5 Years*	Today's date : __/__/__

Health facility (place or vaccination centre) name & address:

Vaccine						*Diluent (if applicable)*			
Name of vaccine	***Date of vaccination***	***Time of vaccination***	Dose (1st, 2nd, etc.)	***Batch /Lot number***	Expiry date	Name of diluent	***Batch /Lot number***	Expiry date	Date and time of reconstitution

Adverse event(s):

☐ Severe local reaction ☐ *>3 days* ☐ *beyond nearest joint*

☐ Seizures ☐ *febrile* ☐ *afebrile*

☐ Abscess
☐ Sepsis
☐ Encephalopathy
☐ Toxic shock syndrome
☐ Thrombocytopenia
☐ Anaphylaxis
☐ Fever ≥38°C
☐ Other (specify)..

Date AEFI started : __/__/__

Time __ __:__ __

Describe AEFI (Signs & Symptoms):

Serious: Yes / No; ➔ If Yes ☐ Death ☐ Life threatening ☐ Persistent or significant disability ☐ Hospitalization ☐ Congenital anomaly
☐ Other important medical event (specify)...

Outcome: ☐ Recovering ☐ Recovered ☐ Recovered with sequelae ☐ Not Recovered ☐ Unknown

☐ Died If Died, date of death : __/__/__ Autopsy done: ☐Yes ☐No ☐Unknown

Past medical history (including history of similar reaction or other allergies), concomitant medication and other relevant information (e.g. other cases). *Use additional sheets if needed:*

First Decision making level to complete:

Investigation needed: ☐ Yes ☐ No	If Yes, date investigation planned : __/__/__

National level to complete:

Date report received at National level __/__/__	AEFI worldwide unique ID :
Comments:	

***Compulsory field**

APPENDIX

Description of elements in the AEFI reporting form (revised Jan 2016)

	Reporting element	Description
	AEFI reporting ID number	Unique number assigned to the AEFI case as per the national guidelines
Patient identifier	*Patient's Name	The name of the patient or initials as decided by the country
	*Patient's full Address	Geographic location of the case (address), please try to provide landmarks
	Telephone	Number to contact to provide or receive additional information
	Sex	Male or Female
	*Date of birth	Date** patient was born
	Age at onset	If date of birth is not known, this may be considered as first alternative
	Age Group at onset	If date of birth and age at onset is not known, this may be considered as second alternative
Reporter details	*Reporter's Name	Name of person who has reported this AEFI to the healthcare system and also completed this form
	Institution	The place where the reporter is working or is affiliated to
	Designation & Department	Reporter's designation and his/her section of work
	Address	Reporters full address - Please add the name of the country here as well
	Telephone	Reporter's phone number
	E-mail	Reporter's e-mail address
	Date patient notified event to health system	The date** when the event was first brought to the notice of the healthcare system
	Today's date	Date** when the report was compiled by the reporter (this can be different from the date of notification (above))
Details of vaccination, vaccine(s) and diluent(s)	Vaccination centre or place of vaccination - name & address	Name and address of the place where the child received the vaccine - provide details (e.g. mobile clinic, home etc.)
	*Name of vaccine	The vaccine that is suspected to have caused the AEFI (provide brand name, if possible)
	Name (of other vaccines)	Other vaccines that were administered at the same time (provide brand name, if possible)
	*Date of vaccination	Date** when the vaccine was administered
	*Time of vaccination	Time** when vaccine was administered - try to be as accurate as possible
	*Batch/Lot number (of vaccine)	Batch number/lot number of each of the vaccines mentioned above
	Dose (1st, 2nd, etc.)	Dose number of the vaccine for the vaccinee e.g. 2nd dose of DTP or 5th Dose of OPV etc.
	Expiry date	The date** of expiry for each vaccine
	*Batch/Lot number (of diluent)	The batch/lot number of diluent (if applicable)
	Expiry date (of diluent)	The date** of expiry of the diluent
	Time of reconstitution	Time when the vaccine was reconstituted with the diluent
Adverse event(s)	*Adverse event(s)	The details of the events suspected to be caused by immunization. Multiple events can occur in a single patient. They need to be documented here
	Date & Time AEFI started	Date** and time** the event was first noticed
	Describe AEFI (Signs & Symptoms)	Description of the events in chronological order
	*Serious: Yes / No	If the case is serious, mark "Yes" and indicate one or several options: Death, Life threatening, Persistent or significant disability, Hospitalization, Congenital anomaly or Other important medical event that may jeopardize the patient or may require intervention to prevent one of the outcomes mentioned here
	*Outcome	Outcome of the reaction(s). Indicate status of the patient at the time of reporting: Recovering, Recovered, Recovered with sequelae, Not Recovered, Unknown or Died
	Died	Provide date of death and details of autopsy, if available
	Past medical history	Please include history of similar reaction or other allergies, concomitant medication and other relevant information (e.g. other cases in the locality or among those vaccinated)
Response	First Decision making level to complete	This section has to be completed by the decision maker for a detailed field AEFI investigation.
	Investigation needed	Decision on detailed field AEFI investigation.
	Date investigation planned	Date** when detailed investigation (including field investigation) is planned to start.
	National level to complete	This section has to be completed by the National level to decide on the next steps.
	Date report received at National level	Date** this report was received at the National level
	AEFI worldwide unique ID	Unique ID number (e.g. regulatory authority's case report number) for the AEFI case automatically generated for electronic transmission from National level to International level
	Comments	Please add additional details that will help with processing this report. Please include other documents as attachments, if necessary

* Compulsory field — Items marked with an asterix (*) have to be completed

** Please use the local convention for the format e.g. DD/MM/YY or MM/DD/YY or YY/MM/DD, for time use a 12 or 24 hours format

APPENDIX - 5

Suspected ADR Form - CIOMS

The globally recognized CIOMS I form is a harmonized template for reporting suspected drug-related adverse reactions by regulatory bodies and the pharmaceutical industry. The sections include coded patient demographics, detailed information on suspected medications, comprehensive adverse event descriptions (including medical outcomes), relevant dates, and the identity of the reporter. The CIOMS form is designed to facilitate international sharing and regulatory review, enabling prompt identification and investigation of serious or unexpected ADR trends.

APPENDIX

CIOMS FORM

SUSPECT ADVERSE REACTION REPORT

I. REACTION INFORMATION

1. PATIENT INITIALS (first, last)	1a. COUNTRY	2. DATE OF BIRTH			2a. AGE	3. SEX	4-6 REACTION ONSET			8-12 CHECK ALL APPROPRIATE TO ADVERSE REACTION
		Day	Month	Year	Years		Day	Month	Year	
7 + 13 DESCRIBE REACTION(S) (including relevant tests/lab data)										☐ PATIENT DIED ☐ INVOLVED OR PROLONGED INPATIENT HOSPITALISATION ☐ INVOLVED PERSISTENCE OR SIGNIFICANT DISABILITY OR INCAPACITY ☐ LIFE THREATENING

II. SUSPECT DRUG(S) INFORMATION

14. SUSPECT DRUG(S) (include generic name)		20 DID REACTION ABATE AFTER STOPPING DRUG? ☐ YES ☐ NO ☐ NA
15. DAILY DOSE(S)	16. ROUTE(S) OF ADMINISTRATION	21. DID REACTION REAPPEAR AFTER REINTRODUCTION? ☐ YES ☐ NO ☐ NA
17. INDICATION(S) FOR USE		
18. THERAPY DATES (from/to)	19. THERAPY DURATION	

III. CONCOMITANT DRUG(S) AND HISTORY

22. CONCOMITANT DRUG(S) AND DATES OF ADMINISTRATION (exclude those used to treat reaction)
23. OTHER RELEVANT HISTORY (e.g. diagnostics, allergics, pregnancy with last month of period, etc.)

IV. MANUFACTURER INFORMATION

24a. NAME AND ADDRESS OF MANUFACTURER		
	24b. MFR CONTROL NO.	
24c. DATE RECEIVED BY MANUFACTURER	24d. REPORT SOURCE ☐ STUDY ☐ LITERATURE ☐ HEALTH PROFESSIONAL	
DATE OF THIS REPORT	25a. REPORT TYPE ☐ INITIAL ☐ FOLLOWUP	